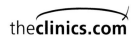

DENTAL CLINICS

OF NORTH AMERICA

Tissue Engineering

GUEST EDITOR
Franklin García-Godoy, DDS, MS

April 2006 • Volume 50 • Number 2

SAUNDERS

An Imprint of Elsevier, Inc.
PHILADELPHIA LONDON TORONTO MONTREAL SYDNEY TOKYO

W.B. SAUNDERS COMPANY
A Division of Elsevier Inc.

Elsevier Inc. • 1600 John F. Kennedy Boulevard • Suite 1800 • Philadelphia, Pennsylvania 19103-2899

http://www.dental.theclinics.com

THE DENTAL CLINICS OF NORTH AMERICA	Volume 50, Number 2
April 2006	**ISSN 0011-8532**
Editor: John Vassallo	**ISBN 1-4160-3573-7**

Reprints: For copies of 100 or more, of articles in this publication, please contact the Commercial Reprints Department, Elsevier Inc., 360 Park Avenue South, New York, New York, 10010-1710. Tel.: (212) 633-3813, Fax: (212) 462-1935, email: reprints@elsevier.com.

The ideas and opinions expressed in *The Dental Clinics of North America* do not necessarily reflect those of the Publisher. The Publisher does not assume any responsibility for any injury and/or damage to persons or property arising out of or related to any use of the material contained in this periodical. The reader is advised to check the appropriate medical literature and the product information currently provided by the manufacturer of each drug to be administered to verify the dosage, the method and duration of administration, or contraindications. It is the responsibility of the treating physician or other health care professional, relying on independent experience and knowledge of the patient, to determine drug dosages and the best treatment for the patient. Mention of any product in this issue should not be construed as endorsement by the contributors, editors, or the Publisher of the product or manufacturers' claims.

The Dental Clinics of North America (ISSN 0011-8532) is published quarterly by W.B. Saunders, 360 Park Avenue South, New York, NY 10010-1710. Months of publication are January, April, July, and October. Business and Editorial Offices: 1600 John F. Kennedy Boulevard, Suite 1800, Philadelphia, PA 19103-2899. Accounting and Circulation Offices: 6277 Sea Harbor Drive, Orlando, FL 32887-4800. Periodicals postage paid at New York, NY and additional mailing offices. Subscription prices are $155.00 per year (US individuals), $255.00 per year (US institutions), $75.00 per year (US students), $185.00 per year (Canadian individuals), $315.00 per year (Canadian institutions), $105.00 per year (Canadian students), $210.00 per year (international individuals), $315.00 per year (international institutions), and $105.00 per year (international students). International air speed delivery is included in all *Clinics* subscription prices. All prices are subject to change without notice. **POSTMASTER:** Send address changes to *The Dental Clinics of North America*, Elsevier Periodicals Customer Service, 6277 Sea Harbor Drive, Orlando, FL 32887-4800. Customer Service: 1-800-654-2452 (US). From outside of the US, call 1-407-345-4000.

The Dental Clinics of North America is covered in *Index Medicus, Current Contents/Clinical Medicine, ISI/BIOMED* and *Clinahl*.

Printed in the United States of America.

GUEST EDITOR

FRANKLIN GARCÍA-GODOY, DDS, MS, Professor and Associate Dean for Research, College of Dental Medicine, Nova Southeastern University, Fort Lauderdale, Florida

CONTRIBUTORS

ZACHARY R. ABRAMSON, BS, Center for Craniofacial Regeneration and Department of Periodontics and Oral Medicine, University of Michigan, Ann Arbor, Michigan

HARU ABUKAWA, DDS, PhD, Research Associate, Department of Oral and Maxillofacial Surgery, Massachusetts General Hospital, Boston, Massachusetts

MAILIKAI ABULIKEMU, MD, MSc, Research Technologist, Department of Oral and Maxillofacial Surgery, Massachusetts General Hospital, Boston, Massachusetts

BRUCE J. BAUM, DMD, PhD, Gene Therapy and Therapeutics Branch, National Institute of Dental and Craniofacial Research, National Institutes of Health, Department of Health and Human Services, Bethesda, Maryland

MIREILLE BONNEFOIX, Laboratoire de Réparation et Remodelage des Tissus Oro-Faciaux, Groupe Matrices Extracellulaires et Biomineralisations, Faculté de Chirurgie Dentaire, Université René Descartes, Montrouge, France

BARBARA D. BOYAN, PhD, Professor of Biomedical Engineering, Georgia Institute of Technology, Atlanta, Georgia

HÉLÈNE CHARDIN, Laboratoire de Réparation et Remodelage des Tissus Oro-Faciaux, Groupe Matrices Extracellulaires et Biomineralisations, Faculté de Chirurgie Dentaire, Université René Descartes, Montrouge, France

ANA P. COTRIM, DDS, PhD, Gene Therapy and Therapeutics Branch, National Institute of Dental and Craniofacial Research, National Institutes of Health, Department of Health and Human Services, Bethesda, Maryland

PAMELA DENBESTEN, Growth and Development Department, University of California at San Francisco, San Francisco, California

JAMES C. EARTHMAN, PhD, Departments of Biomedical Engineering, Chemical Engineering and Materials Science, and Orthopaedic Surgery, University of California, Irvine, California

FRANKLIN GARCÍA-GODOY, DDS, MS, Professor and Associate Dean for Research, College of Dental Medicine, Nova Southeastern University, Fort Lauderdale, Florida

WILLIAM V. GIANNOBILE, DDS, DMedSc, Center for Craniofacial Regeneration and Department of Periodontics and Oral Medicine; Department of Biomedical Engineering, College of Engineering, University of Michigan; and Michigan Center for Oral Health Research, University of Michigan Clinical Center, Ann Arbor, Michigan

MICHEL GOLDBERG, Laboratoire de Réparation et Remodelage des Tissus Oro-Faciaux, Groupe Matrices Extracellulaires et Biominéralisations, Faculté de Chirurgie Dentaire, Université René Descartes, Montrouge, France

NADEGE JEGAT, Laboratoire de Réparation et Remodelage des Tissus Oro-Faciaux, Groupe Matrices Extracellulaires et Biominéralisations, Faculté de Chirurgie Dentaire, Université René Descartes, Montrouge, France

QIMING JIN, DDS, PhD, Center for Craniofacial Regeneration and Department of Periodontics and Oral Medicine, University of Michigan, Ann Arbor, Michigan

LEONARD B. KABAN, DMD, MD, W.C. Walter Guralnick Professor and Chief of Service, Department of Oral and Maxillofacial Surgery, Massachusetts General Hospital, Boston, Massachusetts

SALLY LACERDA-PINHEIRO, Laboratoire de Réparation et Remodelage des Tissus Oro-Faciaux, Groupe Matrices Extracellulaires et Biominéralisations, Faculté de Chirurgie Dentaire, Université René Descartes, Montrouge; and Laboratoire de Differenciation Cellulaire et Prions, Villejuif, France

JEREMY LEAF, BA, Research Student, Department of Oral and Maxillofacial Surgery, Massachusetts General Hospital, Boston, Massachusetts

YONG LI, PhD, Department of Chemical Engineering and Materials Science, University of California, Irvine, California

MICHAEL T. LONGAKER, MD, MBA, Deane P. and Louise Mitchell Professor of Surgery, Division of Plastic and Reconstructive Surgery, Department of Surgery; and Deputy Director, Institute for Stem Cell Biology and Regenerative Medicine, Stanford University School of Medicine, Stanford, California

FUMI MINESHIBA, DDS, PhD, Gene Therapy and Therapeutics Branch, National Institute of Dental and Craniofacial Research, National Institutes of Health, Department of Health and Human Services, Bethesda, Maryland

PETER E. MURRAY, PhD, Assistant Professor, Director of Oral Biology, College of Dental Medicine, Nova Southeastern University, Fort Lauderdale, Florida

RANDALL P. NACAMULI, MD, Postdoctoral Research Fellow, Department of Surgery, Stanford University School of Medicine, Stanford, California

TAKA NAKAHARA, DDS, PhD, Assistant Professor, Section of Developmental and Regenerative Dentistry, School of Life Dentistry at Tokyo, The Nippon Dental University, Tokyo, Japan

MARIA PAPADAKI, DMD, MD, AO-ASIF Clinical Research Fellow, Department of Oral and Maxillofacial Surgery, Massachusetts General Hospital, Boston, Massachusetts

ANNE POLIARD, Laboratoire de Differenciation Cellulaire et Prions, Villejuif, France

FABIENNE PRIAM, Laboratoire de Réparation et Remodelage des Tissus Oro-Faciaux, Groupe Matrices Extracellulaires et Biomineralisations, Faculté de Chirurgie Dentaire, Université René Descartes, Montrouge, France

CHRISTOPH A. RAMSEIER, DMD, Center for Craniofacial Regeneration and Department of Periodontics and Oral Medicine, University of Michigan; and Michigan Center for Oral Health Research, University of Michigan Clinical Center, Ann Arbor, Michigan

DON M. RANLY, DDS, PhD, Director, Dental Technology Center, Georgia Tech Research Institute, Georgia Institute of Technology, Atlanta, Georgia

YUVAL SAMUNI, DMD, PhD, Gene Therapy and Therapeutics Branch, National Institute of Dental and Craniofacial Research, National Institutes of Health, Department of Health and Human Services, Bethesda, Maryland

ZVI SCHWARTZ, DMD, PhD, Professor of Biomedical Engineering, Georgia Institute of Technology, Atlanta, Georgia; and Professor of Periodontics, Hebrew University, Hadassah Faculty of Dental Medicine, Jerusalem, Israel

DOMINIQUE SEPTIER, Laboratoire de Réparation et Remodelage des Tissus Oro-Faciaux, Groupe Matrices Extracellulaires et Biomineralisations, Faculté de Chirurgie Dentaire, Université René Descartes, Montrouge, France

CHERILYN G. SHEETS, DDS, Newport Coast Oral-Facial Institute, Newport Beach, California

NGAMPIS SIX, Laboratoire de Réparation et Remodelage des Tissus Oro-Faciaux, Groupe Matrices Extracellulaires et Biomineralisations, Faculté de Chirurgie Dentaire, Université René Descartes, Montrouge, France

TAKAYUKI SUGITO, DDS, PhD, Gene Therapy and Therapeutics Branch, National Institute of Dental and Craniofacial Research, National Institutes of Health, Department of Health and Human Services, Bethesda, Maryland

KEVIN TOMPKINS, Department of Cell and Molecular Biology, Northwestern University Medical School, Chicago, Illinois

MARIA J. TROULIS, DDS, MSc, Associate Professor and Director of Minimally Invasive Oral and Maxillofacial Surgery, Department of Oral and Maxillofacial Surgery, Massachusetts General Hospital, Boston, Massachusetts

JOSEPH P. VACANTI, MD, John Homans Professor of Surgery and Chief of Pediatric Surgery, Department of Pediatric Surgery, Massachusetts General Hospital; and Director, Laboratory for Tissue Engineering and Organ Fabrication, Massachusetts General Hospital, Boston, Massachusetts

LINDSEY R. VanSCHOIACK, MS, Department of Biomedical Engineering, University of California, Irvine, California

ARTHUR VEIS, Department of Cell and Molecular Biology, Northwestern University Medical School, Chicago, Illinois

DERRICK C. WAN, MD, Resident, Department of Surgery, University of California—San Francisco School of Medicine, San Francisco; and Postdoctoral Research Fellow, Department of Surgery, Stanford University School of Medicine, Stanford, California

JEAN C. WU, DDS, Newport Coast Oral-Facial Institute, Newport Beach, California

PAMELA C. YELICK, PhD, Department of Cytokine Biology, The Forsyth Institute; and Department of Oral Biology, Harvard School of Dental Medicine, Boston, Massachusetts

CONTENTS

> Salivary glands have proven to be unusual but valuable target sites for multiple clinical gene transfer applications. Access to salivary glands for gene transfer is easy. Multiple studies in animal models have yielded proofs of concept for novel treatments for damaged salivary glands following therapeutic irradiation, in Sjögren's syndrome, and for gene therapeutics systemically by way of the bloodstream and locally in the oral cavity and upper gastrointestinal tract.

> Repair and reconstruction of the craniofacial skeleton represents a significant biomedical burden, with thousands of procedures performed annually secondary to injuries and congenital malformations. Given the multitude of current approaches, the need for more effective strategies to repair these bone deficits is apparent. This article explores two major modalities for craniofacial bone tissue engineering: distraction osteogenesis and cellular based therapies. Current understanding of the guiding principles for each of these modalities is elaborated on along with the knowledge gained from clinical and investigative studies. By laying this foundation, future directions for craniofacial distraction and cell-based bone engineering have emerged with great promise for the advancement of clinical practice.

Reconstructive Materials and Bone Tissue Engineering in Implant Dentistry

Periodontal function for natural teeth and dental implants depends strongly on the mechanical integrity of the bone in the maxilla and mandible. Ongoing healthy bone remodeling around a natural tooth or implant is critical for longevity. Chemical factors that influence bone remodeling have been explored with the goal of enhancing the growth and maintenance of good quality bone. Less, but increasing, effort has been directed at understanding mechanical signals and factors, including those affected by implant/prosthesis materials that transmit loads directly to the surrounding bone. This article reviews research on the effects of synthetic materials and resulting mechanical stimuli on bone tissue engineering in dentistry.

There has been significant advancement in the field of periodontal tissue engineering over the past decade for the repair of tooth-supporting structures. Although encouraging results for periodontal tissue regeneration have been found in numerous clinical investigations using recombinant growth factors, limitations exist with topical protein delivery. Newer approaches seek to develop methodologies that optimize growth factor targeting to maximize the therapeutic outcome of periodontal regenerative procedures. Genetic approaches in periodontal tissue engineering show early progress in achieving delivery of growth factor genes, such as platelet-derived growth factor or bone morphogenetic protein, to periodontal lesions. Ongoing investigations in ex vivo and in vivo gene transfer to periodontia seek to examine the extent of the potential effects in stimulating periodontal tissue engineering.

This article focuses on recent advances in the regeneration of periodontium using tissue engineering and examines new technologies that will lead to further advances in periodontal therapy. The various advantages and drawbacks of protein-based, cell-based, and genetic-engineering approaches are evaluated. The debate between those who aim to regenerate periodontal tissues and researchers who have focused on the reconstitution of structural elements of the teeth is examined. The isolation of human dental stem cells from deciduous and adult wisdom teeth might hold the key to allowing the replacement of teeth and the regeneration of supporting tissue. The combination of scientific research, following on from advances in other fields, with clinical research in dentistry could yield a solution to the debilitating and widespread problem of periodontitis.

> After implantation in the exposed pulp, some molecules of the dentin extracellular matrix induce the formation of a reparative dentinal bridge in the coronal pulp. In some cases, total occlusion of the root canal also is observed. This is the case for bone sialoprotein, bone morphogenetic protein-7, Dentonin (a fragment from matrix extracellular phosphoglycoprotein), and two small amelogenin gene splice products (A+4 and A−4). Cells implicated in the reparative process are recruited, proliferate, and differentiate into osteoblast-like and odontoblast-like cells. The same results may be obtained by direct implantation of odontoblast progenitor cell into the pulp.

> Ideally, root canal therapy involves the removal of diseased pulp tissues and permanent replacement with healthy pulp to revitalize teeth. Rather than placing implants, the ideal solution is to grow new replacement teeth. Success rates of implants and endodontic treatments can exceed 90%, which presents a formidable challenge to tissue engineering researchers to ensure that future dental treatments are even more successful. The purpose of this article is to explain how tissue engineering can be used to create replacement teeth. The science of tissue engineering has evolved from growing simple tissues in cell culture incubators to a multistep process. Although the problems of introducing tissue engineering therapies as part of routine dental treatments are substantial, the potential benefits are equally ground breaking.

FORTHCOMING ISSUES

RECENT ISSUES

GOAL STATEMENT

The goal of the *Dental Clinics of North America* is to keep practicing dentists up to date with current clinical practice in dentistry by providing timely articles reviewing the state of the art in dental care.

ACCREDITATION

The *Dental Clinics of North America* are planned and implemented in accordance with the ADA CERP Recognition Standards and Procedures through the joint sponsorship of the University of Virginia School of Medicine and Elsevier.

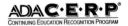 **The University of Virginia School of Medicine is an ADA CERP Recognized Provider.**

Dentists participating in this learning activity may earn up to 15 ADA CERP credits per issue or a maximum of 60 credits per year. Credits awarded may not apply toward license renewal in all states. It is the responsibility of each participant to verify the requirements of their state licensing board.

ADA CERP credit can be earned by reading the text material, taking the CME examination online at http://www.theclinics.com/home/cme, and completing the evaluation. After taking the test, you will be required to review any and all incorrect answers. Following completion of the test and evaluation, your credit will be awarded, and you may print your certificate.

FACULTY DISCLOSURE/CONFLICT OF INTEREST

The University of Virginia School of Medicine, as an ACCME accredited provider, endorses and strives to comply with the Accreditation Council for Continuing Medical Education (ACCME) Standards of Commercial Support, Commonwealth of Virginia statutes, University of Virginia policies and procedures, and associated federal and private regulations and guidelines on the need for disclosure and monitoring of proprietary and financial interests that may affect the scientific integrity and balance of content delivered in continuing medical education activities under our auspices.

The University of Virginia School of Medicine requires that all CME activities accredited through this institution be developed independently and be scientifically rigorous, balanced and objective in the presentation/discussion of its content, theories, and practices.

All authors/editors participating in an accredited CME activity are expected to disclose to the readers relevant financial relationships with commercial entities occurring within the past 12 months (such as grants or research support, employee, consultant, stock holder, member of speakers bureau, etc.). The University of Virginia School of Medicine will employ appropriate mechanisms to resolve potential conflicts of interest to maintain the standards of fair and balanced education to the reader. Questions about specific strategies can be directed to the Office of Continuing Medical Education, University of Virginia School of Medicine, Charlottesville, Virginia.

The authors/editors listed below have identified no professional/financial relationships for themselves or their spouses/partners:
Zachary R. Abramson, BS; Haru Abukawa, DDS, PhD; Mailikai Abulikemu, MD, MSc; Bruce J. Baum, DMD, PhD; Mireille Bonnefoix; Hélène Chardin; Ana P. Cotrim, DDS, PhD; Pamela Denbesten, DDS, MS; Franklin García-Godoy, DDS, MS; Michel Goldberg, DDS, DSc; Nadege Jegat; Qiming Jin, DDS, PhD; Leonard B. Kaban, DMD, MD; Sally Lacerdo-Pinheiro; Jeremy Leaf, BA; Yong Li, PhD; Michael T. Longaker, MD, MBA; Fumi Mineshiba, DDS, PhD; Peter E. Murray, PhD; Randall P. Nacamuli, MD; Taka Nakahara, DDS, PhD; Maria E. Papadaki, DDS, MD; Anne Poliard; Fabienne Priam; Christoph A. Ramseier, DMD; Yuval Samuni, DMD, PhD; Zvi Schwartz, DMD, PhD; Dominique Septier; Ngampis Six; Takayuki Sugito, DDS, PhD; Kevin Tompkins; Maria J. Troulis, DDS, MSc; Lindsey R. VanSchoiack, MS; John Vassallo, Acquisitions Editor; Arthur Veis, PhD; Derrick C. Wan, MD; Jean C. Wu, DDS; and Pamela C. Yelick, PhD.

The authors listed below have identified the following professional/financial relationships for themselves:
Barbara D. Boyan, PhD, is a consultant to Dentsply, Institute Straumann, EBI/LP, and MTF; owns stock in Arthrocare, Inc., ISOT, and OsteoBiologies; and is on the Board of Directors for Arthrocare, Inc. and on the Advisory Board for ISOT.
James C. Earthman, PhD, has stock in and holds a patent for Permetrics, LLC.
William V. Giannobile, DDS, DmedSc, is on the Advisory Board for Biomimetic Therapuetics, Inc.
Don M. Ranly, DDS, PhD, owns stock in Arthrocare, Inc., and his wife is on the Board of Directors.
Cherilyn G. Sheets, DDS, has stock in Permetrics, LLC.
Joseph P. Vacanti, MD, is on the Advisory Board and owns stock in Renalworks, Inc. and Bioengineering Networks, Inc.

Disclosure of discussion of non-FDA approved uses for pharmaceutical products and/or medical devices:
The University of Virginia School of Medicine, as an ACCME provider, requires that all faculty presenters identify and disclose any "off label" uses for pharmaceutical and medical device products. The University of Virginia School of Medicine recommends that each physician fully review all the available data on new products or procedures prior to instituting them with patients.

TO ENROLL

To enroll in the Dental Clinics of North America Continuing Medical Education program, call customer service at 1-800-654-2452 or sign up online at http://www.theclinics.com/home/cme. The CME program is available to subscribers for an additional annual fee of $79.00.

THE DENTAL
CLINICS
OF NORTH AMERICA

Dent Clin N Am 50 (2006) xiii–xiv

Preface

Tissue Engineering

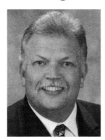

Franklin García-Godoy, DDS, MS
Guest Editor

The age of tissue engineering is upon us. Mankind is advancing beyond the ability to create inanimate objects, toward the capability of replacing and regenerating our own living body tissues. The amalgamation of bioengineering and dentistry will result in an explosion of knowledge that will enhance our understanding of craniofacial development and culminate in a new era in dentistry, enabling us to restore lost tissue function. Tissue engineering is also referred to as "regenerative dentistry," because the goal of tissue engineering is to restore tissue function through the delivery of stem cells, bioactive molecules, or synthetic tissue constructs engineered in the laboratory.

The patient demand for tissue engineering therapies is staggering, both in scope and cost. Each year, $400 billion is spent treating Americans suffering some type of tissue loss or end-stage organ failure. These data include 20,000 organ transplants, 500,000 joint replacements, and hundreds of millions of dental and oral craniofacial procedures ranging from tooth restorations to major reconstruction of facial soft and mineralized tissues. The application of regenerative dentistry in dental clinics can produce wonderful treatments to dramatically improve patients' quality of life. Historically, materials and treatment options have provided the dentist with a limited ability to replace diseased, infected, traumatized, and lost tissues. Looking to the future, advances in bioengineering research are set to unleash the potential of the human genome project and molecular biology into dental practice.

Tissue engineering has become the new frontier in dentistry. A past frontier was the introduction of amalgam restorative materials in the 1830s. By

1845, the American Society of Dental Surgeons, an early professional organization, passed a resolution condemning the use of mercury amalgam as a toxic substance, and expelled members who practiced such use. When used properly, however, the material was long-lasting and relatively easy to manipulate. Eventually, in the late 1890s, largely through the work of Dr. G.V. Black, the "Father of Modern Dentistry," the formulation and proper application of mercury amalgam became better standardized and more successful. The use of dental amalgam has always proven to be controversial and divisive among the general public and dental profession, as it still is today. If we use dental amalgam as a lesson on the controversy of introducing an entirely new type of dental material and treatment, it is easy to speculate that use of tissue engineering in regenerative dentistry will always prove to be controversial.

Controversy surrounding regenerative dentistry is not a bad thing, because it increases scrutiny of its safety, and helps educate the public and profession on its effectiveness and potential disadvantages.

Franklin García-Godoy, DDS, MS
College of Dental Medicine
Nova Southeastern University
3200 South University Drive
Fort Lauderdale, FL 33328, USA

E-mail address: godoy@nsu.nova.edu

ELSEVIER
SAUNDERS

THE DENTAL
CLINICS
OF NORTH AMERICA

Dent Clin N Am 50 (2006) 157–173

Salivary Gland Gene Therapy

Ana P. Cotrim, DDS, PhD, Fumi Mineshiba, DDS, PhD,
Takayuki Sugito, DDS, PhD, Yuval Samuni, DMD, PhD,
Bruce J. Baum, DMD, PhD*

*Gene Therapy and Therapeutics Branch, National Institute of Dental and Craniofacial Research,
National Institutes of Health, Department of Health and Human Services, MSC 1190,
Building 10, Room 1N113, Bethesda, MD 20892-1190, USA*

Why consider gene transfer to salivary glands? Two primary reasons have motivated us. First, no adequate treatment is available for irreversibly damaged salivary glands, such as found in patients receiving therapeutic irradiation (IR) for a head and neck cancer or in patients with the autoimmune exocrinopathy Sjögren's syndrome (SS). Second, salivary glands can produce and secrete large amounts of protein locally to the oral cavity and gastrointestinal (GI) tract or into the bloodstream systemically, making them attractive targets for gene therapeutics (ie, using genes as drugs). This article provides a general background in gene therapy and presents examples, primarily from the authors' laboratory, for clinical salivary gland applications shown feasible in animal models (Table 1). The authors believe that the transfer of genes to salivary glands will prove to be a valuable clinical tool within the next 10 to 20 years. However, and importantly, as of mid-2005, there have been no approved clinical trials involving salivary gland gene transfer.

General strategy

Because of their general organizational structure, salivary glands have some remarkable advantages as target sites for in vivo gene transfer. Almost all epithelial cells in these glands are accessible intraorally in a noninvasive manner. The orifices of the excretory ducts of the major salivary glands (parotid, submandibular/sublingual) exit into the mouth, and are visualized clinically. The delivery of gene transfer vectors in animal models by

---

* Corresponding author.

E-mail address: bbaum@dir.nidcr.nih.gov (B.J. Baum).

0011-8532/06/$ - see front matter. Published by Elsevier Inc.
doi:10.1016/j.cden.2005.11.002

Table 1
Clinical applications of salivary gland gene transfer shown feasible in animal model experiments

Application	Animal model	Transgene	Reference
Irradiation damage	rat, minipig	hAQP1	[1,2]
Sjögren's syndrome	mouse	hIL10, hVIP	[3,4]
Oral-GI tract therapeutics	rat	histatin 3	[5]
Systemic therapeutics	rat, mouse	hGH, hEpo	[6–8]

Abbreviations: hAQP1, human aquaporin-1; hEpo, human erythropoietin; hGH, human growth hormone; hIL10, human interleukin-10; hVIP, human vasoactive intestinal peptide.

cannulation of these ducts, such as done during routine contrast radiography (sialography) of salivary glands, is fairly straightforward to accomplish [9,10]. This approach theoretically allows the vectors to reach the luminal membranes of almost all cells present. Additionally, salivary glands are not critical-for-life organs, and can be removed if an unanticipated adverse effect with considerably less morbidity than would occur with a liver or lung. Also, because human salivary glands have a fibrous capsule, undesirable extra-glandular vector dissemination following intraductal delivery can be minimized.

Genes are transferred into cells by way of vectors, which are critically important variables for success (Table 2). In general terms, two types of gene transfer vectors exist, viral and nonviral. Viral vectors are much more efficient at mediating gene transfer, whereas nonviral vectors pose less of a safety risk. For most of the authors' studies with salivary gland gene transfer one of two viral vectors was used, derived from a serotype 5 adenovirus (Ad5) or a serotype 2 adeno-associated virus (AAV2). Presently, no such thing as a perfect gene transfer vector exists and each of these vectors provides certain advantages [9,10].

Table 2
Key gene transfer vectors tested in salivary glands of animal models

Vector	Animal	Gene expression[b]	Clinical potential[c]	Reference
Plasmid[a]	rat	0.5 +[e]	+	[11,12]
Ad5	many[d]	+ + + +[e]	+ +	[13–16]
AAV2	mouse	+ +[e]	+ + +	[6,17]
FIV	mouse	+ +[e]	+	[18]

[a] Note that plasmids (also sometimes called "naked DNA") are a non-viral means of gene transfer and have been used to deliver genes to salivary glands with the help of cationic lipids.

[b] Relative expression of the transgene on a zero (none) to + + + + (excellent) scale.

[c] Assessment of current relative clinical potential on a zero (none) to + + + + (ideal) scale.

[d] Ad5 vectors have been shown effective for salivary gland gene transfer in mice, rats, minipigs, and non-human primates.

[e] Extent of gene expression is transient for plasmids (1–2 days) and Ad5 vectors (7–14 days), long-lived for AAV2 (>1 year; as long as tested) and FIV (>1 year; as long as tested).

Abbreviations: AAV2, serotype 2 adeno-associated virus; Ad5, serotype 5 adenovirus; FIV, feline immunodeficiency virus.

Ad5 vectors are extremely useful to prove a concept for potential clinical applications. Ad5 vectors lead to transduction of (gene transfer to) virtually all types of epithelial cells in salivary glands, and achieve high levels of gene transfer in vivo, (eg, 20%–35% of the cells) [1,19]. However, Ad5 vectors also can have a negative effect after delivery; they elicit a considerable immune response in salivary glands [13,20,21] as in other tissues. This response, overall, results in high level, but transient, expression of the delivered gene (7–14 days) [19]. Nonetheless, studies by Crystal and colleagues [22,23] have examined the safety of local delivery (to several sites) of low and intermediate doses ($\leq 10^{11}$ viral particles) of Ad5 vectors in humans and concluded that at such doses Ad5 vectors are tolerated well [22,23].

The other viral vector that the authors have used frequently for preclinical, animal model salivary gland gene transfer is derived from AAV2. AAV2 vectors are considerably more difficult to construct than Ad5 vectors, in large part because their biology is less understood than that of Ad5 vectors [9,10]. Use of AAV2 vectors, however, results in much longer transgene expression, with substantially less host immune reactivity, than seen with Ad5 vectors [6,17,24]. Importantly, wild type AAV2 is not associated with any known pathology in humans [25]. Consequently, the authors have decided to use Ad5 vectors routinely to demonstrate conceptual feasibility (though for certain short-term studies, Ad5 vectors may have actual clinical utility) and thereafter use an AAV2 (or in the authors' more recent studies other AAV serotypes) vector if long-term expression is required.

To accomplish actual gene transfer in salivary glands, after suspension in a diluent buffer, vector is infused in a retrograde direction through a cannula placed in Stensen's or Wharton's duct [9]. The volume in which the vector is suspended is optimized for the size and gland type being used [11,14]. This optimization seems to be critical for attaining maximal transgene (the transferred gene) expression and use of a suboptimal volume of suspension buffer leads to marked reductions in the level of transgene product (the encoded protein) produced [14,15]. The optimal volume distends the gland considerably but does not lead to loss of glandular integrity. For example, maximal transgene expression in the murine submandibular gland is achieved with a 50 µL infusate volume, whereas in the rat submandibular gland a 150 to 200 µL infusate is required. In the minipig parotid gland, maximal transgene expression occurs with an infusate volume of 4.0 mL. In the human parotid gland, based on the volume of contrast medium used in sialography, it is estimated that the desirable infusion volume is 1.0 mL.

Irradiation damage: using gene transfer to prevent and repair gland dysfunction

Oral and laryngeal cancer will affect 40,000 Americans in 2005 and more than 350,000 new cases will be diagnosed worldwide [26,27]. The current curative treatment modalities consist of surgery and IR. Salivary glands in the

IR field are damaged severely and, consequently, this results in marked salivary hypofunction in 80% of patients [28–31]. Patients experiencing reduced salivary flow suffer considerable morbidity, including dental caries, mucosal infections, dysphagia, and extensive discomfort. Importantly, the ability to optimize cancer treatments because of relative risks for normal tissue injury has significant implications in oncology, because higher doses of radiation might, in some cases, improve local control and survival [32].

The underlying mechanism of IR-induced injury to the salivary glands is still unknown and somewhat enigmatic. Typically, the most radiosensitive tissues, like hematopoietic progenitor cells, are primitive, undifferentiated cells with a high turnover rate. Conversely, salivary gland cells are highly differentiated epithelial cells and characterized by slow cellular turnover. Yet salivary cells show considerable radiosensitivity, including an acute response to IR resulting in changes in the quantity and composition of saliva within 7 days after beginning radiotherapy [33–37]. Whether direct effects of radiation on the salivary acinar or ductal cells cause radiation damage or if the damage is secondary to injury of adjacent tissue (eg, the fine vascular structures), leading to increased capillary permeability, interstitial edema, and inflammatory cell infiltration is unclear [28–31]. No accepted conventional regimen exists to prevent or correct IR-induced salivary gland damage, and, thus, gene therapy offers a potentially novel way to address this condition. Several genes exist that could be used for these purposes. One example of each is discussed below, for prevention and repair of IR-induced salivary hypofunction.

IR-induced reactive oxygen species (ROS) likely contribute in a significant way to the molecular damage mechanism involved in this condition. When IR interacts with a cell, the resultant transfer of energy increases the intracellular concentration of ROS. These molecules include superoxide ions and hydroxyl radicals. Although these highly reactive free radicals have an extremely short half-life, on the order of 10^{-6} seconds [38], they can have tremendously damaging oxidative effects in the cell. The essential mechanism involved in ROS-mediated damage is the redox (reduction–oxidation) reaction. This reaction involves the transfer of electrons between reactants. Reactants that gain electrons are reduced and those that lose electrons are oxidized. The cellular defense against superoxide ions is the enzyme superoxide dismutase (SOD). At least three forms of this enzyme exists in cells; one found in mitochondria (MnSOD), another in the cytoplasm and nucleus, and a third, an extracellular form [39].

In a series of key studies, involving epithelial tissues generally similar to salivary glands biologically, Greenberger and colleagues [40–47] have advocated a prophylactic role for MnSOD gene transfer in the prevention of IR-induced damage. These investigators demonstrated that pretreatment of mouse lung tissue with the MnSOD gene protected lungs from the acute and chronic sequelae of IR, including radiation pneumonitis and organizing alveolitis and fibrosis [40–43]. This group also has demonstrated that

MnSOD gene transfer could prevent IR-induced esophagitis and oral mucositis in mice in vivo [44–47]. These studies, although not conducted on salivary glands, were conducted on similar tissues and are thus instructive. The MnSOD gene transfer results in a down-regulation of several pro-inflammatory cytokines involved in IR-induced damage. This cytokine down-regulation importantly does not protect orthotopic carcinomas (ie, only normal tissue appears protected from IR damage) [48,49]. Although hydroxyl radicals are likely the primary mediators of oxidative damage to cells, these studies show ample evidence for the benefit of reducing the levels of the superoxide ions for prevention of IR damage to epithelial tissues [50].

The authors' studies have focused on a gene transfer strategy to repair damaged salivary glands following IR. Many surviving former head and neck cancer patients suffer daily from the absence of saliva. To appreciate the rationale behind these studies its important to keep in mind that acinar cells are the only fluid producing cells in the salivary glands, and they are sensitive to IR [51]. Ductal cells, which convey saliva into the mouth, although less sensitive to radiation, are impermeable to water and normally are not considered to be capable of generating salivary fluid flow [9]. Therefore, the loss of acinar cells in a gland will have profound consequences for a patient. Accordingly, the authors have developed a repair strategy designed to permit ductal cells to secrete fluid. The authors hypothesized that by increasing water permeability in surviving cells (presumably mostly ductal) increased fluid secretion would occur. For this purpose the authors and their colleagues constructed a recombinant Ad5 vector (AdhAQP1) encoding the human water channel protein aquaporin-1 (hAQP1) [1]. Water channels allow the rapid movement of water in response to an osmotic gradient across the hydrophobic cell membrane.

Initially, the authors examined rats whose submandibular glands were subjected to a single IR dose of 17.5 or 21 Gy. Three to 4 months after IR, rats were administered a single dose of AdhAQP1, or a control virus, by way of retrograde ductal instillation, and 3 days later, stimulated saliva was collected from all rats. A control virus had no effect on salivary flow and the irradiated rats exhibited marked salivary hypofunction (35% the flow of nonirradiated rats). Conversely, irradiated rats given AdhAQP1 displayed a two- to threefold increase in salivary output above that of irradiated rats given the control virus, approaching salivary flow rates for unirradiated animals treated with the control virus [1].

Subsequently, the atuhors examined the utility of AdhAQP1 for repairing IR damage in nonhuman primates [16]. In this study, one parotid gland of rhesus monkeys (n = 5) was irradiated with a single dose of 10 Gy. This IR dose significantly reduced salivary flow in all monkeys [16]. AdhAQP1 was administered intraductally at 19 weeks after IR and salivary secretion examined 3, 7, and 14 days later. The results, however, were inconsistent, and only two of the four AdhAQP1-treated monkeys displayed increased salivary flow rates compared with a single animal administered an irrelevant virus [16]. Possible reasons for the disparity in results from the rat studies include too few monkeys to permit all desirable control experiments to be performed, an inadequate perfusion of the virus into the primate glands, potential differences between these two animal models in the distribution of viral receptor on the luminal surfaces of gland cells [19], and physiologic differences in the target cells of these two species. However, because of these results, it was unclear if the AdhAQP1 strategy of repairing IR-damaged salivary glands was useful in animals larger than rats.

Therefore, a different, more convenient, and less expensive large animal IR model, the miniature pig (minipig), was developed [15,52]. Using this model, the authors and their colleagues recently evaluated the AdhAQP1-mediated gene transfer strategy after parotid gland IR (20 Gy) [2]. Sixteen weeks following IR, salivation from the targeted gland was decreased by 80%. AdhAQP1 administration resulted in a dose-dependent increase in parotid salivary flow to 80% of pre-IR levels on day 3. A control virus had no significant effect on irradiated minipig parotid flow rates. The effective AdhAQP1 dose was one that leads to comparable transgene expression in murine and minipig salivary glands [15]. Furthermore, 3 days after AdhAQP1 administration little change was observed in clinical chemistry and hematology values in the treated minipigs. Together, these findings demonstrate localized delivery of AdhAQP1 to IR-damaged salivary glands can lead to increases of salivary secretion, without significant general adverse events, in a large animal model, and suggest that the AdhAQP1 strategy may be useful clinically. Based on these results the authors have proposed the use of AdhAQP1 to the FDA for a trial in patients who present with IR-induced parotid hypofunction, and the authors are now developing the clinical protocol for regulatory review.

Sjögren's syndrome

SS is an autoimmune disease, of unclear etiology, characterized by a focal and diffuse lymphoid cell infiltration into the salivary and lacrimal glands (autoimmune exocrinopathy) [53,54]. This chronic immune cell activation leads to reduced secretory function with resulting symptoms of xerostomia (dry mouth) and keratoconjunctivitis sicca (dry eyes). Although SS is characterized by the presence of chronic sialadenitis and dacryoadenitis, many other tissues (eg, the lungs and nervous system) may be involved [53,54]. SS may occur alone (termed primary SS) or develop in association with other autoimmune rheumatic diseases, such as rheumatoid arthritis and systemic lupus erythematosus (termed secondary SS). As in most autoimmune diseases, a sexual dimorphism exists in the prevalence of SS with women affected in greater frequency than men (9:1). One to 2 million persons in the United States are effected.

Although the pathogenesis of SS remains unclear, it has been proposed that a combination of immunologic, genetic, and environmental factors may play important roles in the development of autoimmune reactivity. The glandular lymphocytic infiltrates consist of T cells (up to 80%) and less B cells and plasma cells (20%) [55]. SS is associated with the production of autoantibodies also and these likely reflect B-cell activation and a loss of immune tolerance in the B cell compartment. Several nonorgan specific autoantibodies are important in SS (eg, anti-Ro/SSA, anti-La/SSB, rheumatoid factor, and anti-α-fodrin). Antimuscarinic receptor antibodies seem to be organ-specific autoantibodies that may be important in understanding the pathogenesis of impaired glandular function in SS [56,57].

T helper cell type 1 (Th1) and T helper cell type 2 (Th2) cytokine profiles have been studied in blood, saliva, and salivary gland tissues from patients who have SS [58,59] and from autoimmune mice [60]. Th1 cells produce interleukin (IL)-2, interferon gamma (IFN-γ), and lymphotoxin, all of which are associated with cell-mediated immunity [61]. Th2 cells produce IL-4, IL-5, IL-6, IL-10, and IL-13, which stimulate humoral responses [62]. Cytokines are expressed by lymphocytes infiltrating the salivary glands of patients who have SS. Th2 cytokines are predominant in the early phase of SS, whereas a shift toward Th1 cytokines is associated with advanced lymphocytic infiltration at a later stage of the disease [63].

Apoptotic (cell death) pathways may play important roles for the pathogenesis of SS. For example, Kong and colleagues [64] and Matsumura and colleagues [65] have reported that ductal and acinar cells, and some lymphocytes, undergo apoptosis. In other studies, it has been suggested that perforin and granzyme B from cytotoxic T-lymphocytes are important for the apoptotic pathogenesis of SS [66]. Several generally expressed autoantigens, such as α-fodrin, and tissue-restricted autoantigens, such as the muscarinic receptor isoform 3, which are targeted in SS, are cleaved specifically by granzyme B [67]. Thus, apoptosis plays an important role in the pathogenesis of SS.

At present, treatment of SS is essentially palliative. Artificial salivas are used to improve oral dryness and to prevent dental disease, with minimal success. Pilocarpine and civemilene are muscarinic receptor agonists that are used to stimulate salivary secretions in patients with remaining parenchymal tissue. These treatments help to improve symptoms locally [68], but these are not useful for managing the immune features of SS. Develop new treatment strategies for SS is important. The authors and their colleagues have proposed using local gene transfer for managing the salivary component of SS [3,69].

AAV2 vectors have been used for in vivo gene transfer in various autoimmune diseases, including SS and rheumatoid arthritis. AAV2 vectors can infect dividing and nondividing cells and lead to stable transgene expression. Further, as noted earlier, AAV2 vectors result in a modest host immune response. In aggregate, AAV2 vectors seem to be useful for gene transfer in SS [3,69]. However, a single transgene is difficult to identify as useful for correcting the pathology in SS because the pathogenesis of SS is unclear at present. Based on several immunologic characteristics described earlier, there are immunomodulatory molecules that might be useful for local gene transfer to salivary glands [69]—certain cytokines or factors affecting apoptosis, for example.

Although the roles of individual cytokines in the pathogenesis of SS still have not been established clearly, the proinflammatory cytokines probably stimulate cytotoxic T cell processes within the gland. Previously, the authors' laboratory reported that transfer of the human interleukin (IL)-10 gene into salivary glands using an AAV2 vector was effective in preserving salivary flow and reducing the autoimmune sialadenitis in the nonobese diabetic (NOD) mouse that is a model of SS [3]. IL-10 is a homodimeric cytokine with a wide spectrum of immunosuppressive activities. In these studies, NOD mice were treated with an AAV2 vector encoding human IL-10 or a control protein (β-galactosidase) by retrograde submandibular ductal administration at 8 weeks (early, before onset of sialadenitis), or at 16 weeks (late, after onset of sialadenitis). At 20 weeks, salivary flow rates of early and late hIL-10 gene-treated mice were significantly higher than salivary flow rates of control vector-treated mice. Importantly, inflammatory infiltrates (focus scores) in the submandibular glands were reduced significantly in hIL-10 treated NOD mice [3].

Many recognized inhibitors of apoptosis exist and some may be useful for gene transfer to salivary glands in SS. In the salivary glands of SS patients, Bcl-2 (B-cell leukemia/lymphoma-2) and Bcl-x (B-cell leukemia/lymphoma-x) are expressed preferentially in infiltrating mononuclear cells rather than in the acinar and ductal epithelial cells of minor salivary glands. In contrast, acinar and ductal epithelial cells from SS patients express the X-chromosome–linked inhibitor of apoptosis protein (XIAP), a member of the IAP family that inhibits caspase-7 and caspase-3 activation by blocking cytochrome c-induced activation of pro-caspase-9 [70]. Preventing apoptosis may be possible in salivary gland cells through transfer and overexpression of the XIAP (or some related) gene. The authors' laboratory has begun studies to test this hypothesis.

Because the pathogenesis of SS is not understood at present, these treatment strategies must be considered speculative. However, the results obtained in early studies [3] suggest that a local immunomodulatory strategy for SS may be beneficial, though considerably more animal model study is needed before commencing any clinical testing.

Protein secretion pathways in salivary cells

Although salivary glands are considered to be classic exocrine glands, they can secrete proteins in exocrine (to saliva) and endocrine (to the bloodstream) directions. This characteristic is valuable for the two specific gene therapeutics applications mentioned in earlier discussion (see Table 1) and described below: oral/GI tract and systemic. To appreciate how salivary glands can be employed to use genes encoding secreted proteins as drugs, it is important to understand how proteins are secreted from salivary cells. Studies in animal models show that there are at least two general pathways by which protein secretion occurs in salivary cells: a *constitutive* pathway in which certain proteins are secreted continuously from cells at the rates at which they are synthesized and a *regulated* pathway in which secretory proteins are first stored in vesicles within the cells awaiting an extracellular signal for secretion [71–73]. Typically, in cells all over the body, constitutive pathway secretion occurs in a random manner directionally (ie, with an equal probability of the protein crossing all membrane surfaces in a cell), whereas regulated pathway secretion occurs in highly differentiated cells and in a directional manner [71]. In salivary glands, protein secretion by way of the regulated pathway goes across the apical membrane into the forming saliva, whereas most constitutive pathway protein secretion occurs across the basolateral membranes (the largest membrane surface in epithelial cells) in an endocrine manner toward the interstitium and bloodstream [72,74]. Proteins secreted by way of these two different pathways are sorted or segregated in the trans-Golgi network soon after they are synthesized. This sorting is based on specific amino acid sequences of the protein that in effect form a "zip code" directing the cell to deliver them in one or the other manner [75–77]. Classic cell biological studies by Kelly and colleagues [71,78] in the 1980s showed that regulated and constitutive pathway proteins from one cell type are handled in a similar manner when expressed in other cell types.

Because of these unique protein chemical and cell biological characteristics, the transfer of genes encoding proteins secreted by way of the regulated or constitutive pathway can lead to therapeutic proteins being secreted into saliva for delivery to the oral cavity and upper GI tract or into the bloodstream for systemic delivery. The notion of endocrine secretion by salivary glands was suggested as early as the 1950s [79–81], and subsequently described numerous times, eg, a parotid hormone in pigs [82] and glucagon in several species (rat, mouse, rabbit, human) [83]. However, despite accumulating evidence, a role for endocrine secretion in salivary gland physiology is neither widely recognized nor appreciated [84,85].

The authors' laboratory has shown numerous proofs of concept for the secretion of transgenic proteins by way of these two pathways in experimental animals. For example, growth hormone (GH), an endocrine protein normally secreted into the bloodstream by way of the regulated pathway in anterior pituitary somatotrophs, is secreted from salivary glands into saliva [7,72]. Conversely, erythropoietin (Epo), which is secreted by way of the constitutive pathway by kidney epithelial cells, is secreted by this same pathway from salivary cells leading to its' secretion primarily into the bloodstream [6,8]. The former presents a significant but not insurmountable problem for using salivary glands as a surrogate endocrine gland to correct a deficiency in GH or other regulated pathway proteins (ie, GH secreted into saliva is wasted therapeutically) [86]. However, salivary glands should be useful readily as a therapeutic site for correcting deficiencies in constitutive pathway secretory proteins, such as occur in patients with Epo-responsive anemias as a result of chronic renal failure [6]. As is described below, salivary glands can serve as endogenous bioreactors making therapeutic proteins for exocrine (oral/GI tract) and endocrine (systemic) purposes while using classical pharmacologic principles.

Oral/gastrointestinal tract gene therapeutics

Salivary glands are particularly useful target sites for the delivery of therapeutic genes encoding exocrine proteins for use pharmacologically in the oral cavity and the upper GI tract. Saliva continuously covers these tissues and salivary glands normally secrete into saliva many physiologically beneficial proteins that help maintain tissue integrity [87]. Unfortunately, few studies have examined potential salivary gland exocrine gene-therapeutic applications. Early experiments from the authors' own laboratory showed that transgenic proteins could be secreted at significant levels into saliva for therapeutic purposes. Specifically, these studies showed that transfer of the gene for histatin 3, an anticandidal peptide that normally is found in the saliva of old-world primates and humans, could be expressed in rat salivary glands following gene transfer with an Ad5 vector [5]. Clinically, oral mucosal candidiasis is a common opportunistic infection seen in immunosuppresed patients, and its' management is increasingly difficult with the appearance of drug (eg, azole derivatives)-resistant candidal species. The transgenic histatin 3 produced experimentally in rat saliva was effective in killing azole-resistant Candida albicans [5].

Many other naturally occurring antimicrobial peptides exist that might be useful clinically against antibiotic resistant microorganisms, including the defensins and magainins [88,89]. Although these peptides seem useful therapeutically, concern exists because of their potential toxicity with systemic use [90]. However, this toxicity is unlikely a concern with oral/GI tract gene therapeutics because of the concentrated local bioavailability. This subject is ripe for investigation, particularly because of the morbidity from emerging antibiotic resistant bacteria in the oropharyngeal region [91].

A second potential application for local oral/GI tract gene therapeutics is to promote mucosal wound healing. Severe mucosal ulcerations (eg, in patients who have Bechet's syndrome) or in patients receiving cancer treatment (radiation or chemotherapy), are painful, and clinically difficult to manage [92]. In various protein-therapeutic studies, certain growth factors (eg, epidermal growth factor, keratinocyte growth factor) and cytokines (eg, interleukin-11) improve mucosal wound healing [93–95]. However, to be useful therapeutically, the proteins must be applied to mucosal tissues reasonably often and in fairly high concentrations [93]. Conversely, a gene transfer approach could provide continuous local expression of the protein after salivary gland delivery and theoretically be more effective and less expensive. Indeed, it seems that therapeutically necessary concentrations of transgenic secreted proteins in saliva can be achieved following salivary gland gene transfer [5,96].

An important concern for all gene therapeutics (oral/GI tract and systemic) applications, however, is that almost all vectors used for preclinical studies, and all vectors thus far used clinically, lead to the continuous production of the encoded therapeutic proteins [97]. This production may be desirable for some situations, but it is unlikely to be suitable generally. Transgene expression ideally should be regulated, leading to expression of the therapeutic protein as clinically required [97,98]. Although many regulatory systems have been used in preclinical studies, none has yet been approved for clinical use. The rapamycin inducible system [97,98] has been used to control the expression level of a model exocrine protein secreted from salivary glands [96]. By varying the time and dose of rapamycin, tight control of protein expression can be obtained in saliva, with no detectable transgenic protein expression in the absence of the drug. Furthermore, regulation occurred repeatedly over a 2-week period, consistent with the timecourse required in typical conventional therapy for oral infections and ulcers. Certainly, some type of regulation controlling the production of the transgenic protein is essential for the wide general use of salivary glands, or other tissues, for gene therapeutics.

Systemic gene therapeutics

Salivary glands at present are considered potentially excellent targets for gene therapeutics applications in many monogenetic, single endocrine protein deficiency disorders [6,8,84]. Because salivary glands exhibit the constitutive and regulated secretory pathways, they can be used for conveying both types of expressed transgenic secretory proteins [9,72]. As discussed earlier, transgene products in salivary glands continue to use their normal physiologic secretion routes. Proteins that are secreted constitutively in their primary site of production continue to use this route when expressed as a transgene product in salivary glands, and such proteins are predominantly secreted into the bloodstream (ie, in an endocrine manner). Thus, salivary glands may be useful especially as a surrogate endocrine gland for certain diseases in which the deficient protein is normally secreted by way of the constitutive pathway [8].

In 1996, the authors' laboratory reported the first unequivocal demonstration of the secretion of a transgene product from salivary glands into the bloodstream [99]. Human α1-antitrypsin (hα1AT), which is normally secreted in the liver by way of the constitutive pathway, was encoded in an Ad5 vector and delivered to rat submandibular glands. The levels of hα1AT in the bloodstream were four- to fivefold greater than in the saliva [99]. More recently, the authors' laboratory has studied endocrine secretion from salivary glands using a transgene encoding human Epo (hEpo) [6,8].

Physiologically, as discussed above, hEpo is secreted by way of the constitutive pathway. Using an AAV2 vector encoding hEpo, the authors observed stable production of hEpo from mouse salivary glands and its secretion into the bloodstream for more than 1 year, along with associated elevations in hematocrit values [6,8]. The salivary hEpo levels in these studies were 10% of those in the serum. Using various transgenes encoding proteins secreted by the constitutive pathway, it seems that salivary glands readily can achieve circulating levels of transgene products up to 5 ng/mL. Such levels are therapeutically adequate for treating an Epo-responsive anemia but not for treating emphysema caused by a deficiency of $\alpha 1AT$, where levels of greater than 100 µg/ml are required.

As discussed above, administration of vectors encoding GH to salivary glands leads to secretion of GH mainly into saliva; 10 to 20 fold higher levels than that found in the bloodstream. Nonetheless, the GH levels in serum can be sufficient therapeutically [7,8,86]. High levels of GH are produced by salivary cells, saturating entry into the regulated pathway with the excess GH being secreted by way of a constitutive route into the bloodstream. However, because most of the GH produced is being secreted into saliva, it is therapeutically inefficient. In order for salivary glands to be useful as a gene transfer target site for systemically required regulated pathway proteins, such as GH, or other neuroendocrine hormones, some redirection of this type of secretory protein is needed. The authors' laboratory has addressed this concern by using two strategies. With the first approach, studies have tried to alter the specific sorting signal for human GH (hGH) entry into the regulated pathway, so that instead most hGH would exit the salivary cells by the constitutive pathway [100]. This strategy has yielded modest success, likely because the exact sorting signal for hGH is not fully known [100]. With the other strategy, studies have used hydroxychloroquine (HCQ; Plaquenil), a commonly used antimalarial and antirheumatic drug. HCQ disrupts regulated pathway sorting by alkalinizing transport vesicles in the trans-Golgi network, resulting in a mis-sorting of hGH [86]. HCQ treatment in rats leads to a considerable shift in hGH secretion from salivary glands by way of the constitutive pathway, yielding hGH serum levels ∼30 times those required therapeutically. Although both strategies have shown utility in animal studies, considerably more research is required before any human clinical testing.

Summary

Salivary glands have proven to be unusual but valuable target sites for multiple clinical gene transfer applications. Access to salivary glands for gene transfer is easy, and multiple studies in animal models have yielded proofs of concept for novel treatments for damaged salivary glands following therapeutic IR, in SS, and for gene therapeutics systemically by way of the bloodstream and locally in the oral cavity and upper GI tract.

Acknowledgments

The authors thank Drs. Jane Atkinson and Aaron Palmon for their helpful comments on an earlier draft of this manuscript.

References

[1] Delporte C, O'Connell BC, He X, et al. Increased fluid secretion after adenoviral-mediated transfer of the aquaporin-1 cDNA to irradiated rat salivary glands. Proc Natl Acad Sci USA 1997;94:3268–73.

[2] Shan Z, Li J, Zheng C, et al. Increased fluid secretion after adenoviral-mediated transfer of the human aquaporin-1 cDNA to irradiated miniature pig parotid glands. Mol Ther 2005; 11:444–51.

[3] Kok MR, Yamano S, Lodde BM, et al. Local adeno-associated virus-mediated interleukin 10 gene transfer has disease-modifying effects in a murine model of Sjögren's syndrome. Hum Gene Ther 2003;14:1605–18.

[4] Lodde BM, Mineshiba F, Wang J, et al. Effect of human vasoactive intestinal peptide gene transfer in a murine model of Sjogren's syndrome. Ann Rheum Dis 2005 Jun 23 [Epub ahead of print].

[5] O'Connell BC, Xu T, Walsh TJ, et al. Transfer of a gene encoding the anticandidal protein histatin 3 to salivary glands. Hum Gene Ther 1996;7:2255–61.

[6] Voutetakis A, Kok MR, Zheng C, et al. Re-engineered salivary glands are stable endogenous bioreactors for systemic gene therapeutics. Proc Natl Acad Sci USA 2004;101:3053–8.

[7] He X, Goldsmith CM, Marmary Y, et al. Systemic action of human growth hormone following adenovirus-mediated gene transfer to rat submandibular glands. Gene Ther 1998;5: 537–41.

[8] Voutetakis A, Bossis I, Kok MR, et al. Salivary glands as a potential gene transfer target for gene therapeutics of some monogenetic endocrine disorders. J Endocrinol 2005;185:363–72.

[9] Baum BJ, Wellner RB, Zheng C. Gene transfer to salivary glands. Int Rev Cytol 2002;213: 93–146.

[10] Baum BJ, Goldsmith CM, Kok MR, et al. Advances in vector-mediated gene transfer. Immunol Lett 2003;90:145–9.

[11] Baccaglini L, Hoque ATMS, Wellner RB, et al. Cationic liposome-mediated gene transfer to rat salivary epithelial cells in vitro and in vivo. J Gene Med 2001;3:82–90.

[12] Goldfine ID, German MS, Tseng HC, et al. The endocrine secretion of human insulin and growth hormone by exocrine glands of the gastrointestinal tract. Nat Biotechnol 1997;15: 1378–82.

[13] Kagami H, Atkinson JC, Michalek SM, et al. Repetitive adenovirus administration to the parotid gland: role of immunological barriers and induction of oral tolerance. Hum Gene Ther 1998;9:305–13.

[14] Wang S, Baum BJ, Yamano S, et al. Adenoviral-mediated gene transfer to mouse salivary glands. J Dent Res 2000;79:701–8.

[15] Li J, Zheng C, Zhang X, et al. Developing a convenient large animal model for gene transfer to salivary glands in vivo. J Gene Med 2004;6:55–63.

[16] O'Connell AC, Baccaglini L, Fox PC, et al. Safety and efficacy of adenovirus-mediated transfer of the human aquaporin-1 cDNA to irradiated parotid glands of non-human primates. Cancer Gene Ther 1999;6:505–13.

[17] Yamano S, Huang LY, Ding C, et al. Recombinant adeno-associated virus serotype 2 vectors mediate stable interleukin 10 secretion from salivary glands into the bloodstream. Hum Gene Ther 2002;13:287–98.

[18] Shai E, Palmon A, Panet A, et al. Prolonged transgene expression in murine salivary glands following non-primate lentiviral vector transduction. Mol Ther 2005;12:137–43.

[19] Delporte C, Redman RS, Baum BJ. Relationship between the cellular distribution of the alpha (v), beta3/5 integrins and adenoviral infection in salivary glands. Lab Invest 1997; 77:167–73.

[20] Adesanya MR, Redman RS, Baum BJ, et al. Immediate inflammatory responses to adenovirus-mediated gene transfer in rat salivary glands. Hum Gene Ther 1996;7:1085–93.

[21] Wang S, Baum BJ, Kagami H, et al. Effect of clodronate on macrophage depletion and adenoviral-mediated transgene expression in salivary glands. J Oral Pathol Med 1999;28: 145–51.

[22] Harvey B-G, Maroni J, O'Donoghue KA, et al. Safety of local delivery of low- and intermediate-dose adenovirus gene transfer vectors to individuals with a spectrum of comorbid conditions. Hum Gene Ther 2002;13:15–63.

[23] Crystal RG, Harvey BG, Wisnivesky JP, et al. Analysis of risk factors for local delivery of low- and intermediate-dose adenovirus gene transfer vectors to individuals with a spectrum of comorbid conditions. Hum Gene Ther 2002;13:65–100.

[24] Kok MR, Voutetakis A, Yamano S, et al. Immune responses following salivary gland administration of recombinant adeno-associated virus serotype 2 vectors. J Gene Med 2005;7:432–41.

[25] Kay MA, Glorioso JC, Naldini L. Viral vectors for gene therapy: the art of turning infectious agents into vehicles of therapeutics. Nat Med 2001;7:33–40.

[26] The Oral Cancer Foundation. Oral cancer facts. Available at: http://www. oralcancerfoundation.org/. Accessed June 2005.

[27] Day GL. Cancer rates and risks—NIH; NCI—online publication—from the Epidemiology and Extramural Programs Branch, Division of Cancer Etiology, National Cancer Institute. Available at: http://seer.cancer.gov/publications/raterisk/risks175.html. Accessed June 2005.

[28] Grdina DJ, Murley JS, Kataoka Y. Radioprotectants: current status and new directions. Oncology 2002;63:2–10.

[29] Vissink A, Jansma J, Spijkervet FK, et al. Oral sequelae of head and neck radiotherapy. Crit Rev Oral Biol Med 2003;14:199–212.

[30] Vissink A, Burlage FR, Spijkervet FK, et al. Prevention and treatment of the consequences of head and neck radiotherapy. Crit Rev Oral Biol Med 2003;14:213–25.

[31] Nagler RM, Baum BJ. Prophylactic treatment reduces the severity of xerostomia following irradiation therapy for oral cavity cancer. Arch Otolaryngol Head Neck Surg 2003;129: 247–50.

[32] Anscher MS, Chen L, Rabbani Z, et al. Recent progress in defining mechanisms and potential targets for prevention of normal tissue injury after radiation therapy. Int J Radiat Oncol Biol Phys 2005;62:255–9.

[33] Vissink A, Kalicharan D, S-Gravenmade EJ, et al. Acute irradiation effects on morphology and function of rat submandibular glands. J Oral Pathol Med 1991;20:449–56.

[34] Taylor SE, Miller EG. Preemptive pharmacologic intervention in radiation-induced salivary dysfunction. Proc Soc Exp Biol Med 1999;221:14–26.

[35] O'Connell AC. Natural history and prevention of radiation injury. Adv Dent Res 2000;14: 57–61.

[36] Burlage FR, Coppes RP, Meertens H, et al. Parotid and submandibular/sublingual salivary flow during high dose radiotherapy. Radiother Oncol 2001;61:271–4.

[37] Nagler RM. The enigmatic mechanism of irradiation-induced damage to the major salivary glands. Oral Dis 2002;8:141–6.

[38] Halliwell B, Gutteridge JM. Role of free radicals and catalytic metal ions in human disease: an overview. Methods Enzymol 1990;186:1–85.

[39] Vitolo JM, Baum BJ. The use of gene transfer for the protection and repair of salivary glands. Oral Dis 2002;8:183–91.

[40] Epperly M, Bray J, Kraeger S, et al. Prevention of late effects of irradiation lung damage by manganese superoxide dismutase gene therapy. Gene Ther 1998;5:196–208.

[41] Epperly MW, Bray JA, Esocobar P, et al. Overexpression of the human manganese super-oxide dismutase (MnSOD) transgene in subclones of murine hematopoietic progenitor cell line 32D cl 3 decreases irradiation-induced apoptosis but does not alter G2/M or G1/S phase cell cycle arrest. Radiat Oncol Investig 1999;7:331–42.

[42] Epperly MW, Defilippi S, Sikora C, et al. Intratracheal injection of manganese superoxide dismutase (MnSOD) plasmid/liposomes protects normal lung but not orthotopic tumors from irradiation. Gene Ther 2000;7:1011–8.

[43] Carpenter M, Epperly MW, Agarwal A, et al. Inhalation delivery of manganese super-oxide dismutase-plasmid/liposomes protects the murine lung from irradiation damage. Gene Ther 2005;12:685–93.

[44] Stickle RL, Epperly MW, Klein E, et al. Prevention of irradiation-induced esophagitis by plasmid/liposome delivery of the human manganese superoxide dismutase transgene. Radiat Oncol Investig 1999;7:204–17.

[45] Epperly MW, Defilippi S, Sikora C, et al. Radioprotection of lung and esophagus by over-expression of the human manganese superoxide dismutase transgene. Mil Med 2002;167: 71–3.

[46] Epperly MW, Carpenter M, Agarwal A, et al. Intraoral manganese superoxide dismutase-plasmid/liposome (MnSOD-PL) radioprotective gene therapy decreases ionizing irradia-tion-induced murine mucosal cell cycling and apoptosis. In Vivo 2004;18:401–10.

[47] Guo H, Seixas-Silva JA Jr, Epperly MW, et al. Prevention of radiation-induced oral cavity mucositis by plasmid/liposome delivery of the human manganese superoxide dismutase (SOD2) transgene. Radiat Res 2003;159:361–70.

[48] Epperly MW, Travis EL, Sikora C, et al. Manganese [correction of Magnesium] superoxide dismutase (MnSOD) plasmid/liposome pulmonary radioprotective gene therapy: modula-tion of irradiation-induced mRNA for IL-I, TNF-alpha, and TGF-beta correlates with delay of organizing alveolitis/fibrosis. Biol Blood Marrow Transplant 1999;5:204–14.

[49] Guo H, Epperly MW, Bernarding M, et al. Manganese superoxide dismutase-plasmid/lipo-some (MnSOD-PL) intratracheal gene therapy reduction of irradiation-induced inflamma-tory cytokines does not protect orthotopic Lewis lung carcinomas. In Vivo 2003;17:13–21.

[50] Epperly MW, Sikora CA, DeFilippi SJ, et al. Manganese superoxide dismutase (SOD2) inhibits radiation-induced apoptosis by stabilization of the mitochondrial membrane. Radiat Res 2002;157:568–77.

[51] Nagler RM. Effects of head and neck radiotherapy on major salivary glands–animal studies and human implications. In Vivo 2003;17:369–75.

[52] Li J, Shan Z, Ou G, et al. Structural and functional characteristics of irradiation damage to parotid glands in the miniature pig. Int J Rad Oncol Biol Phys 2005;62(5):1510–6.

[53] Bloch KJ, Buchanan WW, Wohl MJ, et al. Sjögren's syndrome. A clinical, pathological, and serological study of sixty-two cases. Medicine (Baltimore) 1965;44:187–231.

[54] Fox RI, Michelson P, Casiano CA, et al. Sjögren's syndrome. Clin Dermatol 2000;18: 589–600.

[55] Jonsson R, Haga H-J, Gordon TP. Sjögren's syndrome. In: Koopman WJ, editor. Arthritis and allied conditions: a textbook of rheumatology. 14th edition. Philadelphia: Lippincott, Williams & Wilkins; 2001. p. 1736–59.

[56] Bacman S, Sterin-Borda L, Camusso JJ, et al. Circulating antibodies against rat parotid gland M3 muscarinic receptors in primary Sjögren's syndrome. Clin Exp Immunol 1996; 104:454–9.

[57] Nguyen KH, Brayer J, Cha S, et al. Evidence for antimuscarinic acetylcholine receptor antibody-mediated secretory dysfunction in nod mice. Arthritis Rheum 2000;43:2297–306.

[58] Garcic-Carrasco M, Font J, Filella X, et al. Circulating levels of Th1/Th2 cytokines in patients with primary Sjögren's syndrome: correlation with clinical and immunological features. Clin Exp Rheumatol 2001;19:411–5.

[59] Streckfus C, Bigler L, Navazesh M, et al. Cytokine concentrations in stimulated whole sa-liva among patients with primary Sjögren's syndrome, secondary Sjögren's syndrome, and

patients with primary Sjögren's syndrome receiving varying doses of interferon for symptomatic treatment of the condition: a preliminary study. Clin Oral Investig 2001;5:133–5.

[60] van Blokland SC, Versnel MA. Pathogenesis of Sjögren's syndrome: characteristics of different mouse models for autoimmune exocrinopathy. Clin Immunol 2002;103:111–24.

[61] Abbas AK, Murphy KM, Sher A. Functional diversity of helper T lymphocytes. Nature 1996;383:787–93.

[62] Mosmann TR, Coffman RL. TH1 and TH2 cells: different patterns of lymphokine secretion lead to different functional properties. Annu Rev Immunol 1989;7:145–73.

[63] Mitsias DI, Tzioufas AG, Veiopoulou C, et al. The Th1/Th2 cytokine balance changes with the progress of the immunopathological lesion of Sjögren's syndrome. Clin Exp Immunol 2002;128:562–8.

[64] Kong L, Ogawa N, McGuff HS, et al. Bcl-2 family expression in salivary glands from patients with primary Sjögren's syndrome: involvement of Bax in salivary gland destruction. Clin Immunol Immunopathol 1998;88:133–41.

[65] Matsumura R, Umemiya K, Kagami M, et al. Glandular and extraglandular expression of the Fas-Fas ligand and apoptosis in patients with Sjögren's syndrome. Clin Exp Rheumatol 1998;16:561–8.

[66] Polihronis M, Tapinos NI, Theocharis SE, et al. Modes of epithelial cell death and repair in Sjögren's syndrome (SS). Clin Exp Immunol 1998;114:485–90.

[67] Nagaraju K, Cox A, Casciola-Rosen L, et al. Novel fragments of the Sjögren's syndrome autoantigens alpha-fodrin and type 3 muscarinic acetylcholine receptor generated during cytotoxic lymphocyte granule-induced cell death. Arthritis Rheum 2001;44:2376–86.

[68] Nusair S, Rubinow A. The use of oral pilocarpine in xerostomia and Sjögren's syndrome. Semin Arthritis Rheum 1999;28:360–7.

[69] Kok MR, Baum BJ, Tak PP, et al. Use of localised gene transfer to develop new treatment strategies for the salivary component of Sjogren's syndrome. Ann Rheum Dis 2003;62:1038–46.

[70] Nakamura H, Kawakami A, Yamasaki S, et al. Expression and function of X chromosome-linked inhibitor of apoptosis protein in Sjögren's syndrome. Lab Invest 2000;80:1421–7.

[71] Kelly RB. Pathways of protein secretion in eukaryotes. Science 1985;230:25–32.

[72] Baum BJ, Berkman ME, Marmary Y, et al. Polarized secretion of transgene products from salivary glands in vivo. Hum Gene Ther 1999;10:2789–97.

[73] Isenman L, Liebeow C, Rothman S. The endocrine secretion of mammalian digestive enzymes by exocrine glands. Am J Physiol 1999;276:E223–32.

[74] Castle D, Castle A. Intracellular transport and secretion of salivary proteins. Crit Rev Oral Biol Med 1998;9:4–22.

[75] Loh YP, Maldonado A, Zhang C. Mechanisms of sorting proopiomelanocortin and proenkephalin to the regulated secretory pathway of neuroendocrine cells. Ann N Y Acad Sci 2002;971:416–25.

[76] Gorr S-U, Jain RK, Kuehn U, et al. Compartive sorting of neuroendocrine secretory proteins: a search for common ground in the mosaic sortin models and mechanisms. Mol Cell Endocrinol 2001;172:1–6.

[77] Feliciangeli S, Kitabgi P, Bidard JN. The role of dibasic residues in prohormone sorting to the regulated secretory pathway. J Biol Chem 2001;276:6140–50.

[78] Burgess T, Kelly RB. Constitutive and regulated secretion of protein. Annu Rev Cell Biol 1987;3:243–93.

[79] Ogata T. The internal secretion of salivary glands. Endocrinol Jpn 1955;2:247–61.

[80] Ishikawa H. Endocrine function of the salivary glands. Allerg Asthma (Leipz) 1956;2:42–3.

[81] Godlowski ZZ, Calandra JC. Salivary glands as endocrine organs. J Appl Physiol 1960;15:101–5.

[82] Leonara J, Steinman RR. Evidence suggesting the existence of a hypothalamic-parotid gland endocrine axis. Endocrinology 1968;83:807–15.

[83] Lawrence AM, Tan S, Hojvaat S, et al. Salivary gland hyperglycemic factor: an extra-pancreatic source of glucagon-like material. Science 1977;195:70–2.

[84] Baum BJ, Voutetakis A, Wang J. Salivary glands: novel target sites for gene therapeutics. Trends Mol Med 2004;10:585–90.

[85] Zufferey R, Aebischer P. Salivary glands and gene therapy: the mouth waters. Gene Ther 2004;11:1425–6.

[86] Hoque ATMS, Baccaglini L, Baum BJ. Hydroxychloroquine enhances the endocrine secretion of adenovirus-directed growth hormone from rat submandibular gland in vivo. Hum Gene Ther 2001;12:1333–41.

[87] Van Nieuw Amerongen A, Veerman EC. Saliva—the defender of the oral cavity. Oral Dis 2002;8:12–22.

[88] Maisetta G, Batoni G, Esin S, et al. Activity of human β-defensin 3 alone or combined with other antimicrobial agents against oral bacteria. Antimicrob Agents Chemother 2003;47: 3349–51.

[89] Zasloff M. Innate immunity, antimicrobial peptides, and protection of the oral cavity. Lancet 2002;360:1116–7.

[90] Gura T. Innate immunity: ancient system gets new respect. Science 2001;291:2068–71.

[91] Martin JM, Green M, Barbadora KA, et al. Erythromycin-resistant group A streptococci in schoolchildren in Pittsburgh. N Engl J Med 2002;364:1200–6.

[92] Sonis ST, Peterson DE, McGuire DB, et al. Prevention of mucositis in cancer patients. J Natl Cancer Inst Monogr 2001;29:1–2.

[93] Palomino A, Hernandez-Bernal F, Haedo W, et al. A multicenter, randomized, double-blind clinical trial examining the effect of oral human recombinant epidermal growth factor on the healing of duodenal ulcers. Scand J Gastroenterol 2000;35:1016–22.

[94] Dorr W, Noack R, Spekl K, et al. Modification of oral mucositis by keratinocyte growth factor: single radiation exposure. Int J Radiat Biol 2001;77:341–7.

[95] Sonis ST, Peterson RL, Edwards LJ, et al. Defining the mechanisms of action of interleukin-11 on the progression of radiation-induced oral mucositis in hamsters. Oral Oncol 2000;36: 373–81.

[96] Wang J, Voutetakis A, Zheng C, et al. Rapamycin control of exocrine protein levels in saliva after adenoviral vector-mediated gene transfer. Gene Ther 2004;11:729–33.

[97] Rivera VM, Clackson T, Natesan S, et al. A humanized system for pharmacological control of gene expression. Nat Med 1996;2:1028–32.

[98] Clackson T. Regulated gene expression systems. Gene Ther 2000;7:120–5.

[99] Kagami H, O'Connell BC, Baum BJ. Evidence for the systemic delivery of a transgene product from salivary gland. Hum Gene Ther 1996;7:2177–84.

[100] Wang J, Cawley NX, Voutetakis A, et al. Partial redirection of transgenic human growth hormone secretion from rat salivary glands. Hum Gene Ther 2005;16:571–83.

ELSEVIER
SAUNDERS

THE DENTAL
CLINICS
OF NORTH AMERICA

Dent Clin N Am 50 (2006) 175–190

Craniofacial Bone Tissue Engineering

Derrick C. Wan, MD, Randall P. Nacamuli, MD,
Michael T. Longaker, MD, MBA*

*Stanford University School of Medicine, 257 Campus Drive West,
Stanford, CA 94305-5148, USA*

Since the turn of the millennium, the annual growth in United States health care expenditure has increasingly outpaced the annual growth in gross domestic product by ever-increasing margins [1]. Current expenditures exceed $1.5 trillion, with unabated demand, burgeoning costs, and an aging population contributing to this predicament. Data from the United States Healthcare Utilization Project revealed that over 1 million skeletal-related procedures were performed in 2002, with 16,338 craniotomies/craniectomies and 32,043 post-traumatic facial reconstructions accounting for over $585 million in medical care [2]. Extending these procedures to include the correction of congenital craniofacial anomalies and malformations only serves to further underscore the biomedical burden associated with the treatment of skeletal defects.

Large bone defects resulting from trauma, tumor resection, nonunion of fractures, and congenital malformations are common clinical problems in craniofacial surgery, which have proven difficult to remedy. Current surgical techniques have used, in various combinations, autogenous, allogeneic, and prosthetic materials to achieve bone reconstruction [3]. However, the multitude of dissimilar solutions currently in practice highlights the fact that an ideal solution has yet to be defined. Autogenous bone grafting generally has yielded favorable results, but this practice is limited by donor-site morbidity and the amount of bone that may be harvested [4,5]. In situations where insufficient autogenous bone exists, use of allogeneic bone may also be used. This approach, however, is also beset with a multitude of concerns, chief among which include infection, immunologic rejection,

This work was supported by National Institutes of Health grants R01 DE13194 and R01 DE14526 and the OAK Foundation (to M.T. Longaker) and the Ethicon-Society of University Surgeons Research Fellowship (to D.C. Wan).

* Corresponding author.
E-mail address: Longaker@stanford.edu (M.T. Longaker).

and graft-versus-host disease [5]. Alternative materials have therefore been developed to assist in bone reconstruction, with metal alloys, glass, plaster of paris, polymethylmethacrylate, and, more recently, biodegradable scaffolds all being investigated [3,6,7]. Discouragingly, none of these modalities have yet to prove a consummate tool for craniofacial bone reconstruction.

By combining decades of clinical experience with recent studies in molecular, cell, and developmental biology, however, the field of bone tissue engineering has rapidly become a practical approach to the treatment of many craniofacial skeletal defects. Mechanical-based (distraction osteogenesis) and cell-based (multipotent mesenchymal cell) modalities have garnered particular attention not only from an investigational stand point but also from their present-day clinical applications [8,9]. Since its general introduction over 50 years ago, distraction osteogenesis has revolutionized the treatment of many congenital hypoplasias afflicting children [10,11]. As a form of endogenous tissue engineering, distraction osteogenesis has spread rapidly throughout the field of craniofacial reconstruction and is currently the treatment of choice for several midface and mandibular deformities [12–14]. Like distraction osteogenesis, regenerative medicine also has the potential to transform the field of craniofacial skeletal repair through a cell-based approach to engineer bone. At its core, regenerative medicine incorporates the use of multipotent building blocks combined with molecular and environmental cues for the repair of damaged or diseased tissue. Recent investigations have focused upon the post natal mesenchymal stromal cell population that has been demonstrated to possess the ability to differentiate down multiple lineages in appropriate environments [15]. As studies continue to define the true nature of these cells, their potential for clinical application already has been demonstrated in the report of a calvarial defect reconstruction from Germany in 2004 [9].

Considering the large biomedical burden skeletal reconstruction comprises, distraction osteogenesis and cell-based tissue engineering increasingly will become critical modalities for craniofacial bone reconstruction. Both modalities carry the potential for generation of novel bone without the attendant limitations of current allogeneic and prosthetic strategies. This article focuses on these two significant paradigms for craniofacial bone tissue engineering and present emerging knowledge from recent investigations to elucidate the biologic underpinnings of these processes.

Distraction osteogenesis

Reconstruction of skeletal hypoplasias involving the mandible, maxilla, midface, orbits, and cranial vault continues to present a significant challenge to contemporary craniofacial surgeons. Children who present with bony insufficiencies often suffer from a host of disabilities ranging from severe airway compromise to malocclusion and a dysfunctional bite. Traditional approaches at reconstruction using osteotomies and bone grafting can be associated with unsatisfactory outcomes and significant short- and long-term morbidities. Since the adoption of distraction osteogenesis to the correction of craniofacial skeletal hypoplasias, however, more favorable results have been obtained and this modality rapidly has become the treatment of choice for several midface and mandibular deficiencies.

Distraction osteogenesis is a powerful form of endogenous tissue engineering, promoting bone formation through the gradual separation of osteogenic fronts. Despite its recent application to craniofacial surgery, the fundamental principles of distraction osteogenesis have existed since the early twentieth century [16]. In 1956, Ilizarov [11,17,18] demonstrated this modality could be consistently applied to long bone reconstruction with acceptable morbidity. The first translation to intramembranous bone of the craniofacial skeleton was established in 1972 using a canine model and, in 1989, McCarthy [8] performed the first human mandibular distraction [19]. Since that landmark description, this technique has now become a standard tool for craniofacial surgeons to achieve clinically significant midface and mandibular advancement.

As elaborated by Ilizarov, distraction osteogenesis incorporates rigid fixation with a several day latency period, followed by gradual distraction and stable fixation until radiographic and clinical assessment demonstrates the formation of a robust, mineralized regenerate [11,17,18]. Despite ever increasing experience, however, significant complications nonetheless continue to plague surgeons performing this procedure; overall morbidity rates as high as 35% have been described [20]. Most commonly, soft-tissue infection, osteomyelitis, and pin-tract infection or loosening secondary to daily manipulation of exposed devices have been reported. Patient discomfort and complications related to compliance also contribute to overall morbidity. Lastly, fibrous nonunion, permanent inferior alveolar nerve injury, and relapse of the original condition typically within the first 6 months following distraction remain significant considerations in the postoperative period [20]. In the face of such concerns, however, overall results remain acceptable, with surgeons reporting good or excellent results in over 86% of patients [21,22].

With a goal to further optimize these clinical outcomes and minimize associated complications, recent investigations have endeavored to better characterize the mechanisms guiding successful bone formation in the regenerate. These studies have focused primarily on the mechanobiology and molecular biology of successful osteogenesis during guided distraction. Large animal models, including canine, ovine, and lupine species, have been used traditionally in these investigations to delineate the histologic and ultrastructural changes associated with robust bone deposition [19,23–25]. Studies using such models, though, have been frustrated by animal size, cost, and relative dearth of molecular reagents available. Recent work by Fang and colleagues [26], however, have established a mouse model of mandibular distraction osteogenesis to exploit the wide breadth of molecular reagents, microarray analysis, recent advances in bioluminescent reporting, microcomputed tomography, and perhaps most importantly, transgene constructs available in mice. With the development of this model system, clear advantages arise with regard to cost, scalability, and flexibility for the performance of more detailed investigations to define the fundamental mechanisms behind successful bone deposition in the regenerate.

Mechanobiology

The impact of mechanical environment on bone development and maintenance is central to the study of mechanobiology. Dynamic loading has been shown to be critical for preservation and increase of bone mass in vivo and, on a cellular level, has been found to modulate osteoblast and osteoclast activity [27,28]. Recent studies also have suggested a role for hydrostatic stress and tensile strain in the orchestration of multipotent mesenchymal progenitor cell differentiation into bone, cartilage, and fibrous tissue [29–31]. In addition, cyclic motion and associated shear stress has been shown to accelerate cellular proliferation and callus production [29]. Nonetheless, as the significance of mechanical environment on bone formation is unmistakable, how forces contribute to proper osteogenesis in the distraction regenerate remains a paramount issue to be fully elucidated.

The characterization of resultant stress and strain patterns during distraction is essential to define how mechanical forces ultimately influence guided osteogenesis. By correlating histologic findings with measurements of tensile force, Loboa and colleagues [32] demonstrated the highest rates of bone formation occur during active mandibular distraction, with typical strain ranging between 10% and 12.5% across the regenerate. Measured strain was noted to have a viscoelastic response, reaching highest levels immediately following distraction and gradually declining to less than half the peak level with time [32]. Further work using finite element analysis revealed specific patterns of tensile strain and hydrostatic stress characteristics across the distraction gap. Within the gap itself, mesenchymal tissues were noted to experience moderate hydrostatic stress predictive of bone formation by way of intramembranous ossification. In contrast, mild compressive stress was observed in the periphery, compatible with endochondral ossification around the periosteal edges. These predictions based on finite element analysis remarkably mirror histologic findings in multiple animal models of mandibular distraction, with the appearance of direct bone formation within the distraction gap and cartilaginous intermediates adjacent to osteotomized fronts [26,32].

Having defined a blueprint for the stress engendered during distraction osteogenesis, recent investigations have focused on manipulations of the mechanical environment to accelerate successful bone deposition in the regenerate. Efforts to minimize the protracted course of standard protocols already have raised doubt over the necessity of a latency period, with recent studies demonstrating no significant benefit for delay of distraction [20, 33–35]. Investigations using the ovine and porcine models have exposed no differences in mechanical strength, radiographic appearance, or bone density of the regenerate when latency periods of 4 or 7 days were compared with no latency [34,35]. Furthermore, retrospective studies have revealed similar results in the clinical setting, suggesting the traditional practice of latency–while still observed by most contemporary surgeons–may not be critically important and its reduction or elimination may serve to shorten the total duration of distraction osteogenesis without any detriment to bone deposition [20].

Though reduction of latency can afford a small gain in shortening the overall process of distraction, the greatest gains may conceivably be made by hastening the period of consolidation. Consequently, investigations have focused specifically on callus stimulation to accelerate maturation of the regenerate into mineralized bone. Axial loading in long bone fracture segments already has been shown to increase callus bulk, promote fracture healing, and hasten onset of bony union [36]. Adapting this principle to mandibular distraction, Mofid and colleagues [33] demonstrated cyclic loading of the regenerate during early consolidation to yield increased callus size, cortical density, and mineral apposition rate. Alternatively, callus stimulation has also been achieved through use of pulsed ultrasound, with analogous pro-osteogenic effects seen on bone formation in the distraction gap. The introduction of daily low-intensity ultrasound at a frequency of 1 kHz during mandibular distraction has been shown to accelerate time to completion of consolidation in rabbit models. Whether through cyclic loading or pulsed ultrasound, the notion of callus simulation therefore suggests an appealing approach to enhance bone formation and healing in craniofacial reconstruction. The application of callus stimulation to craniofacial distraction possibly may hasten the period of consolidation and thus minimize overall related patient morbidity. And by integrating this notion with data garnered from mechanical models of environmental stress, novel, more effective distraction protocols may be developed and translated into clinical practice.

Molecular biology

Although investigations have begun to elucidate the complex interplay of forces involved in bone formation during guided distraction, how this ultimately leads to changes at the cellular level to favor osteogenesis remains undefined. How cells respond to exogenous forces and translate these physical signals into a biomolecular cascade resides at the root of current investigations on mechanotransduction. Studies by Banes and colleagues [37] have established that forces can act directly at the cellular level, whether through mechanical-sensitive ion channels, integrin-cytoskeleton machinery, or load-sensitive receptor or nonreceptor tyrosine kinases. Furthermore, a link between the extracellular mechanical environment and intracellular signaling cascade recently has been demonstrated through the localization of focal adhesion kinase protein to regions of bone formation during mandibular distraction [38]. As focal adhesion kinase has been implicated as an intermediary between cell-surface integrins and several MAP kinase cascades, a tangible biologic foundation for the influence of exogenous stress on bone formation has already been established.

With the advent of small animal models for mandibular distraction, significant strides have recently been made in defining the molecular processes regulating de novo bone formation in the regenerate. Studies have demonstrated a potential involvement for several pro-osteogenic cytokines, such as bone morphogenetic proteins (BMPs) and other members of the TGFβ superfamily [39–41]. Analyzing temporospatial expression patterns for BMPs 2, 4, and 7, histologic and immunohistochemical assessment have revealed an upregulation in osteoblasts during mandibular distraction [41]. Chondrocytes, likewise, were found to augment BMP expression particularly during the period of consolidation. Capitalizing on these findings, Ashinoff and colleagues [42] demonstrated that bone formation in the mandibular regenerate could be accelerated by local delivery of BMP-2 during consolidation through an adenoviral vector. By radiographic, histologic, and histomorphometric analyses, a significant increase in bone deposition could be induced, suggesting a biologic modality to enhance clinical distraction outcomes.

Although several investigations have highlighted the significance of BMPs in distraction osteogenesis, other cytokines have likewise gained increasing attention for their potential involvement in bone formation. Using a mouse model of mandibular distraction, Fang and colleagues [26] noted a dramatic rise in VEGF and FGF-2 expression during the period of active distraction. Quantitative real-time RT-PCR analysis revealed a fourfold increase in expression for both of these angiogenic factors relative to acutely lengthened hemimandible controls [26]. Immunohistochemical staining of goat mandibular regenerates have also demonstrated analogous findings, with intense staining for VEGF and FGF-2 during active distraction [43]. Recent studies designed to suppress these angiogenic signals have revealed provocative results, further underscoring the significance of an appropriate biomolecular environment for proper bone formation following mandibular distraction. Through administration of TNP-470, a fumagillin analog which inhibits endothelial cell proliferation and new capillary formation, complete nonunion was observed in all distracted hemimandibles [44–46]. Histologic assessment demonstrated no intramembranous bone formation within the distraction gap or evidence of endochondral bone along the periosteum. With PECAM staining showing no obvious blood vessel formation, the data suggest that direct failure of angiogenesis may, in part, have contributed to the failure of osteogenesis observed [46]. Despite appropriate mechanical signaling, an adequate angiogenic network–through VEGF or FGF-2 signaling–may thus be equally integral to the successful generation of new bone in the distraction gap.

Incorporating data obtained through mechanical investigations with recent findings in cytokine biology, a more lucid picture of the instruments guiding bone formation in distraction osteogenesis has therefore begun to develop. By using knowledge gained from mechanical stimulation and modeling of associated forces combined with manipulations in pro-osteogenic and pro-angiogenic cytokine signaling, a new paradigm for the clinical approach toward craniofacial distraction may emerge presently.

Cellular therapies

Despite the enormous potential for the generation of de novo bone using distraction osteogenesis, this modality nonetheless is limited in craniofacial repair. Some forms of craniosynostosis, certain craniofacial hypoplasias, and injuries secondary to facial trauma present clinical situations in which an approach using guided distraction may not engineer all of the necessary bone. The need for alternative modalities has therefore continued to drive the use of autogenous, allogeneic, and prosthetic materials to reconstruct the craniofacial skeleton [4,6,7,47–52]. As mentioned, however, these strategies are beset by numerous shortcomings, including infection, immunologic rejection, and graft-versus-host disease [51,53]. In addition, donor-site morbidity, in the case of autogenous bone harvest, may be protracted with ambulatory difficulty or chronic pain reported in as high as 51% of patients [54]. With these considerations in mind, researchers have therefore sought to develop novel methods to generate bone in the craniofacial skeleton.

Recent advances in cellular-based tissue engineering have made this a potentially attractive approach for the repair of bony defects given its widespread adaptability. With novel, moldable scaffolds providing specific molecular and environmental niches, the capacity for finely controlled bone formation is readily achievable. Contentious debate, however, has surrounded the identification of an optimal source for osteoprogenitors. Irrespective of this, the promise of tissue engineered bone through cell-based modalities has made this approach ever more appealing for the repair of calvarial and facial defects.

Cell-based approaches

Research has focused intently on defining the consummate cellular building block with which to base therapy for skeletal repair. Several human embryonic stem cell lines have been demonstrated to possess the capacity to differentiate into various tissue types [55]. Considerable controversy, however, has accompanied the study of these embryonic stem cells, with significant political and ethical hurdles encumbering further investigations [56–58]. Although work continues with somatic-cell nuclear transplantation for the generation of genotype predefined pluripotent cell-lines, the therapeutic use of such cells will continue to remain illusory in the foreseeable future [59]. In similar fashion, recent debate has surrounded the clinical application of gene therapy and genetically modified adult cells [60]. Though early enthusiasm for this form of gene therapy has led to the race to develop treatments for genetic and non-genetic-based diseases, adverse outcomes have led to calls for a potential moratorium [60–63].

Over the last decade, the regenerative capacity of postnatal progenitor cells has increasingly emerged making these cells an attractive candidate for use in tissue-engineering applications. Whether these cells represent true pluripotent cells or more committed multipotent or oligopotent progenitors remains to be defined, but their capacity to differentiate into a multitude of cell types has been demonstrated abundantly [15,64–66]. Speculation, however, continues as to how these cells may function in tissue repair. Arguments for and against direct participation in the generation of new tissue or creation of conducive environments for endogenous host cell differentiation have been raised [67,68]. Nonetheless, the procurement and use of these postnatal progenitor cells allows for cellular based tissue engineering to proceed unfettered by the political and ethical concerns surrounding alternative cell sources.

Substantial work has already progressed with these postnatal progenitors, with early studies concentrating on mesenchymal stem cells (MSCs) naturally residing within bone marrow. Several investigators have demonstrated this cell population to contribute to the regeneration of other mesenchymal tissues throughout the body, including bone, cartilage, muscle, ligament, tendon, adipose, and stroma [15,69–71]. Furthermore, using bone marrow aspirates from over 350 human donors, Pittenger and colleagues [15] were able to show lineage specific differentiation of these MSCs into fat, cartilage, and bone under appropriate in vitro culture conditions. Not only did the human bone-marrow-derived MSCs demonstrate ability to extensively proliferate, but these cells also were capable of guided differentiation into multiple cell types, establishing a provocative cell source for potential craniofacial tissue engineering [15].

The concept of critical-sized defect reconstruction using mesenchymal stem cells harvested from bone marrow already has been validated in several animal models [72,73]. Implanting these cells within a fibrin glue construct into 15 mm parietal defects in rabbits, investigators have demonstrated healing and similar cellular integration into surrounding corticocancellous bone when compared with implanted osteoblasts [73]. Mechanical testing of the regenerate revealed equivalent stiffness and strength in defects filled with bone marrow-derived mesenchymal cells or harvested osteoblasts, both of which demonstrated significantly more healing than defects left unfilled [73]. Similar studies have found application of bone marrow-derived MSCs in the reconstruction of orbital defects in pigs [74]. But while great enthusiasm surrounds the use of these cells in craniofacial tissue engineering, several limiting factors have made bone marrow-derived MSCs less attractive. Selective sera and growth factor supplements have been reported by

[55] Thomson JA, et al. Embryonic stem cell lines derived from human blastocysts. Science 1998;282(5391):1145–7.

[56] Weissman IL. Stem cells–scientific, medical, and political issues. N Engl J Med 2002; 346(20):1576–9.

[57] Bahadur G. The moral status of the embryo: the human embryo in the UK Human Fertilisation and Embryology (Research Purposes) Regulation 2001 debate. Reprod Biomed Online 2003;7(1):12–6.

[58] Chin JJ. Ethical issues in stem cell research. Med J Malaysia 2003;58(Suppl A):111–8.

[59] Hwang WS, et al. Patient-specific embryonic stem cells derived from human SCNT blastocysts. Science 2005;308(5729):1777–83.

[60] Dixon N. Cancer scare hits gene cures: a second major setback for medicine's most pioneering treatment has split the scientific community. Could a moratorium do more harm than good? New Sci 2002;176(2364):4–5.

[61] Grilley BJ, Gee AP. Gene transfer: regulatory issues and their impact on the clinical investigator and the good manufacturing production facility. Cytotherapy 2003;5(3): 197–207.

[62] Smith L, Byers JF. Gene therapy in the post-Gelsinger era. Jonas Healthc Law Ethics Regul 2002;4(4):104–10.

[63] Verma IM. A voluntary moratorium? Mol Ther 2003;7(2):141.

[64] Forbes SJ, Poulsom R, Wright NA. Hepatic and renal differentiation from blood-borne stem cells. Gene Ther 2002;9(10):625–30.

[65] Pittenger MF, Mosca JD, McIntosh KR. Human mesenchymal stem cells: progenitor cells for cartilage, bone, fat and stroma. Curr Top Microbiol Immunol 2000;251:3–11.

[66] Zuk PA, et al. Human adipose tissue is a source of multipotent stem cells. Mol Biol Cell 2002;13(12):4279–95.

[67] Wagers AJ, et al. Little evidence for developmental plasticity of adult hematopoietic stem cells. Science 2002;297(5590):2256–9.

[68] Wagers AJ, Weissman IL. Plasticity of adult stem cells. Cell 2004;116(5):639–48.

[69] Prockop DJ. Marrow stromal cells as stem cells for nonhematopoietic tissues. Science 1997; 276(5309):71–4.

[70] Haynesworth SE, Baber MA, Caplan AI. Cell surface antigens on human marrow-derived mesenchymal cells are detected by monoclonal antibodies. Bone 1992;13(1):69–80.

[71] Haynesworth SE, et al. Characterization of cells with osteogenic potential from human marrow. Bone 1992;13(1):81–8.

[72] Schantz JT, et al. Repair of calvarial defects with customized tissue-engineered bone grafts I. Evaluation of osteogenesis in a three-dimensional culture system. Tissue Eng 2003; 9(Suppl 1):S113–26.

[73] Schantz JT, et al. Repair of calvarial defects with customised tissue-engineered bone grafts II. Evaluation of cellular efficiency and efficacy in vivo. Tissue Eng 2003;9(Suppl 1): S127–39.

[74] Rohner D, et al. In vivo efficacy of bone-marrow-coated polycaprolactone scaffolds for the reconstruction of orbital defects in the pig. J Biomed Mater Res B Appl Biomater 2003; 66(2):574–80.

[75] Haynesworth SE, Baber MA, Caplan AI. Cytokine expression by human marrow-derived mesenchymal progenitor cells in vitro: effects of dexamethasone and IL-1 alpha. J Cell Physiol 1996;166(3):585–92.

[76] De Ugarte DA, et al. Comparison of multi-lineage cells from human adipose tissue and bone marrow. Cells Tissues Organs 2003;174(3):101–9.

[77] Mendes SC, et al. Bone tissue-engineered implants using human bone marrow stromal cells: effect of culture conditions and donor age. Tissue Eng 2002;8(6):911–20.

[78] Banfi A, et al. Proliferation kinetics and differentiation potential of ex vivo expanded human bone marrow stromal cells: implications for their use in cell therapy. Exp Hematol 2000;28(6):707–15.

[79] Auquier P, et al. Comparison of anxiety, pain and discomfort in two procedures of hematopoietic stem cell collection: leukacytapheresis and bone marrow harvest. Bone Marrow Transplant 1995;16(4):541–7.

[80] Nishimori M, et al. Health-related quality of life of unrelated bone marrow donors in Japan. Blood 2002;99(6):1995–2001.

[81] Bergman RJ, et al. Age-related changes in osteogenic stem cells in mice. J Bone Miner Res 1996;11(5):568–77.

[82] Stenderup K, et al. Aging is associated with decreased maximal life span and accelerated senescence of bone marrow stromal cells. Bone 2003;33(6):919–26.

[83] Stenderup K, et al. Aged human bone marrow stromal cells maintaining bone forming capacity in vivo evaluated using an improved method of visualization. Biogerontology 2004; 5(2):107–18.

[84] Mueller SM, Glowacki J. Age-related decline in the osteogenic potential of human bone marrow cells cultured in three-dimensional collagen sponges. J Cell Biochem 2001;82(4): 583–90.

[85] Zuk PA, et al. Multilineage cells from human adipose tissue: implications for cell-based therapies. Tissue Eng 2001;7(2):211–28.

[86] Batinic D, et al. Relationship between differing volumes of bone marrow aspirates and their cellular composition. Bone Marrow Transplant 1990;6(2):103–7.

[87] Bacigalupo A, et al. Bone marrow harvest for marrow transplantation: effect of multiple small (2 ml) or large (20 ml) aspirates. Bone Marrow Transplant 1992;9(6):467–70.

[88] Shi Y, et al. The osteogenic potential of adipose-derived mesenchymal cells is maintained with aging. Plast Reconstr Surg 2005;116(6):1686–96.

[89] Lee JA, et al. Biological alchemy: engineering bone and fat from fat-derived stem cells. Ann Plast Surg 2003;50(6):610–7.

[90] Hicok KC, et al. Human adipose-derived adult stem cells produce osteoid in vivo. Tissue Eng 2004;10(3–4):371–80.

[91] Saadeh PB, et al. Repair of a critical size defect in the rat mandible using allogenic type I collagen. J Craniofac Surg 2001;12(6):573–9.

[92] Seol YJ, et al. Chitosan sponges as tissue engineering scaffolds for bone formation. Biotechnol Lett 2004;26(13):1037–41.

[93] Bumgardner JD, et al. Chitosan: potential use as a bioactive coating for orthopaedic and craniofacial/dental implants. J Biomater Sci Polym Ed 2003;14(5):423–38.

[94] Solchaga LA, et al. Treatment of osteochondral defects with autologous bone marrow in a hyaluronan-based delivery vehicle. Tissue Eng 2002;8(2):333–47.

[95] Albee FH. Studies in bone growth: triple CaP as a stimulus to osteogenesis. Ann Surg 1920; 71:32–6.

[96] Schliephake H, et al. Repair of calvarial defects in rats by prefabricated hydroxyapatite cement implants. J Biomed Mater Res 2004;69A(3):382–90.

[97] Blokhuis TJ, et al. Properties of calcium phosphate ceramics in relation to their in vivo behavior. J Trauma 2000;48(1):179–86.

[98] Lanza RP, Langer RS, Vacanti J. Principles of tissue engineering. 2nd edition. San Diego (CA): Academic Press 2000.

[99] Behravesh E, et al. Synthetic biodegradable polymers for orthopedic applications. Clin Orthop Res Relat 1999;(367 Suppl):S118–29.

[100] Kokubo T, Kim HM, Kawashita M. Novel bioactive materials with different mechanical properties. Biomaterials 2003;24(13):2161–75.

[101] Chou YF, et al. The effect of biomimetic apatite structure on osteoblast viability, proliferation, and gene expression. Biomaterials 2005;26(3):285–95.

THE DENTAL
CLINICS
OF NORTH AMERICA

Dent Clin N Am 50 (2006) 191–203

Bioengineered Teeth from Tooth Bud Cells

Pamela C. Yelick, PhD[a,b,]*, Joseph P. Vacanti, MD[c,d]

[a]*Department of Cytokine Biology, The Forsyth Institute, Boston, MA, USA*
[b]*Department of Oral Biology, Harvard School of Dental Medicine, Boston, MA, USA*
[c]*Department of Pediatric Surgery, Massachusetts General Hospital, Boston, MA, USA*
[d]*Laboratory for Tissue Engineering and Organ Fabrication, Massachusetts General Hospital,
Boston, MA, USA*

Prospects for bioengineered dental tissue repair and regeneration therapies

The ability to obtain and manipulate postnatal tissues easily from individuals to generate biologic replacement tooth materials, such as dentin, enamel, and periodontal ligament, or, even better, replace teeth of predetermined size and shape entirely, is extremely valuable. Dental tissues exhibit little to no regenerative capabilities [1]. Small amounts of reparative dentin can be induced to form in response to subtle tooth injury [2–4], and cementum also exhibits limited regenerative capabilities [5]. In contrast, enamel exhibits no regenerative capacity, because progenitor dental epithelial cells that form enamel lose this ability well before tooth eruption [6]. Because individual teeth generally do not last the lifetime of individuals without requiring at least some repair—cavity filling, root canal, crown, or, at worst, extraction—the need for replacement teeth and dental tissue repair therapies is significant. As the close association between oral health, systemic health, and nutrition becomes more apparent [7], the necessity of proper oral health for long-term quality of life becomes more appreciated [8,9].

Exacerbating the nonregenerative nature of natural tooth tissues, a range of circumstances threatens the health and longevity of teeth on a regular

This work was supported by National Institutes of Health/National Institute of Dental and Craniofacial Research grants DE015445, DE016132, and DE016370, the Center for Integration of Medicine and Innovative Technology (CIMIT), Harvard School of Dental Medicine, and The Forsyth Institute.

* Corresponding author. Department of Cytokine Biology, The Forsyth Institute, 140 The Fenway, Boston, MA 02115.

E-mail address: pyelick@forsyth.org (P.C. Yelick).

basis. The risk for sustaining tooth injury is prevalent due to a variety of factors, including injuries obtained in sports and accident-related trauma [10], oral and other cancers, cancer treatment therapies in children and elderly populations [11,12], periodontal disease, and diabetes [13]. In addition, parafunctional habits, such as teeth grinding or clenching, and everyday chewing of foods, including soft foods, such as bread, and, in particular, hard foods, can result in chipped or cracked teeth. The high susceptibility of teeth to damage, combined with the nonregenerative nature of dental tissues, emphasizes the need for replacement tooth therapies. Until the present time, the fields of restorative dentistry and materials sciences have combined efforts to produce a variety of synthetic materials for use in the restoration of damaged dental hard tissues. Although these materials and therapies have proved effective, they do not exhibit the same mechanical and physical properties as naturally formed dentin and enamel. Differences in the physical properties of synthetic versus natural tooth tissues can result in uneven wear of synthetic and natural tooth tissues over time, resulting in unanticipated stresses on opposing and adjacent teeth. The somewhat incompatible physical properties of synthetic and natural tooth tissues can contribute to compromised oral health, which in turn can result in systemic health issues. Oral tissue infections and associated nutritional deficits can lead to imbalances in oral flora populations, eventually contributing to compromised overall health and reduced quality of life [14].

A tissue engineering approach to dental tissue regeneration

Based on recent reports indicating significant progress in bioengineering a variety of adult hard and soft tissues, the authors tested the ability to use a similar approach to bioengineering dental tissues. Using successful techniques of bioengineering neonatal intestine [15,16] and stomach [17], the authors used immature tooth bud tissue, enriched in dental progenitor cells, to seed biodegradable scaffolds that then were implanted in a host animal to provide sufficient vascularization of bioengineered tissues (Fig. 1). When the implants were harvested and analyzed after 25 to 30 weeks of growth, in many instances, the dissociated tooth bud cells had reorganized into what appeared to be small, anatomically correct tooth crowns with rudimentary tooth root structures (Fig. 2). Molecular and cellular analyses of bioengineered tooth tissues generated from pig [18] and rat tooth bud cells [19] demonstrate that developing bioengineered tooth crowns express the same genes and proteins found in naturally formed teeth [20]. The demonstration that a tissue engineering approach could be used to regenerate dental tissues is promising, suggesting that clinically relevant therapies based on this approach could be used to repair or regenerate dental tissues and whole teeth.

The current task is how to perfect tooth tissue engineering techniques, such that bioengineered dental tissues and whole teeth are integrated

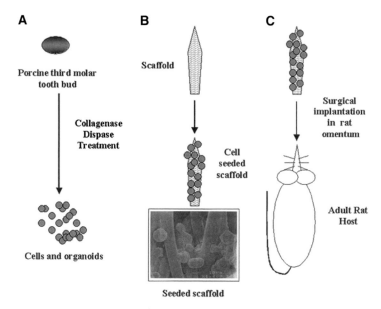

Fig. 1. Omental implant method schematic. Tooth bud cell-seeded scaffolds were implanted into the omenta of adult rat hosts, as diagrammed. (*A*) Tooth buds are dissociated into single-cell suspensions. (*B*) Cells are seeded onto biodegradable scaffolds. (*C*) Cell-seeded scaffolds are implanted into rat hosts.

physically and functionally with pre-existing dental tissues. Ideally, bioengineered dentin and enamel used to repair defects in pre-existing teeth can be integrated seamlessly with pre-existing naturally formed dentin and enamel crystals, eliminating the presence of interface sites susceptible to refracturing. Bioengineered whole teeth would be modeled to occlude with opposing and adjacent teeth properly and anchored to underlying alveolar bone via periodontal ligament tissue to transmit mechanical signals properly, allowing for orthodontic treatments as required. Biologic tooth substitutes would exhibit proper proprioception, facilitating the life of the implant and adjacent and opposing teeth.

Currently, with state-of-the-art techniques and materials for tissue engineering technologies, it is clear that these ambitious goals eventually can be achieved. Before tooth tissue engineering can become a widely practiced, clinically available therapy, however, impediments that are not insignificant must be overcome. Existing challenges in tooth tissue engineering can be classified broadly into two areas: (1) the identification and characterization of suitable dental progenitor cell populations that can be obtained easily and used for autologous tooth tissue engineering practices; and (2) the development of methods to reproducibly manipulate dental progenitor cells to bioengineer dental tissues and whole teeth of predetermined size and shape in a timely fashion. This article describes current efforts and future plans to facilitate the creation of clinically relevant tooth tissue engineering

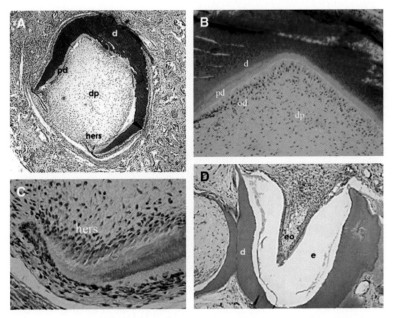

Fig. 2. Bioengineered dental tissues. (*A*) von Kossa staining of sectioned 20-week dental implant reveals bioengineered tooth crown exhibiting distinct pulp and predentin and dentin tissues. High magnification view of bioengineered tooth crown (*B*) and rudimentary Hertwig's epithelial root (hers) structure (*C*). (*D*) 30-week implant contains bioengineered teeth with significant amounts of dentin and enamel. d, dentin; dp, dental pulp; e, enamel; eo, enamel organ; hers, Hertwig's epithelial root sheath; od, odontoblasts; p, pulp; pd, predentin.

methodologies for the repair and regeneration of dental tissues from autologous adult tissues.

Characterization of tooth bud cell populations

The dental progenitor cells used in the authors' initial tooth tissue engineering studies were obtained from immature, unerupted tooth buds isolated from 6-month-old pigs [18] and 4-day postnatal rats [19]. The rationale for using pig and rat teeth at these developmental stages was to obtain tooth bud cell populations enriched in the two types of dental progenitor cells required to form all of the tissues in teeth and supporting periodontal ligament and alveolar bone tissues—epithelial and mesenchymal dental stem cells (DSC). Tooth bud tissues were dissociated enzymatically and mechanically and filtered to remove even small clumps of cells, generating single cell suspensions. The single cell suspensions were plated in vitro and cultured for approximately 1 week to eliminate differentiated cell types that do not survive long term in culture, resulting in enriched postnatal dental progenitor cell populations. Cultured cells then were harvested and seeded onto biodegradable polyester scaffolds, the purpose of which was to provide a support onto which seeded dental progenitor cells—post-natal dental stem cells (PNDSC)—can adhere and orient themselves with respect to each other, allowing for requisite epithelial and mesenchymal dental cell interactions for tooth initiation and development. The cell-seeded scaffolds were grown in the omenta of host animals, an environment conducive to promote vascularization and growth of dental implant tissues.

Early results demonstrated that small tooth crowns formed in pig tooth bud cell-seeded implants grown for approximately 20 to 30 weeks [18] and in rat tooth bud cell-seeded implants grown for approximately 12 weeks [19]. The amount of time required to form bioengineered pig versus rat tooth crowns correlates with the amount of time required for naturally formed pig and rat teeth to develop and, therefore, likely reflects an endogenous developmental program for pig and rat PNDSC that is retained even when whole tooth buds are dissociated into single cell suspensions and cultured in vitro. The ability of PNDSC to retain a dental tissue differentiation program facilitates their use in dental tissue repair and whole tooth tissue engineering applications.

Histologic analyses of bioengineered dental implants reveal that small tooth crowns form throughout the implant. Tooth tissues form initially at the periphery and subsequently in the center of the implant, suggesting that PNDSC migrate from the periphery into the center of the scaffold over time before differentiating into dental tissues [20].

The fact that bioengineered dental tissue implants consist of many small bioengineered tooth crowns, with apparent random orientation, rather than one large bioengineered tooth adopting the size and shape of the scaffold onto which the PNDSC are seeded, reveals insight into certain properties of these cells. Because tooth formation depends on the interactions of two types of dental cells—epithelial and mesenchymal—it is logical to assume that each bioengineered tooth crown forms at sites within the scaffold to which both types of PNDSC are able to migrate, attain cell-cell contact, and initiate and maintain the reiterative and reciprocal growth factor signaling cascades leading to tooth development [21]. Another assumption is that only a subset of the total cell population seeded onto the scaffold is able to initiate or maintain a successful tooth development program, because small tooth crowns are scattered throughout the implant and generally form as discrete structures. These observations are consistent with the extensive literature documenting the heterogeneity of tooth bud tissues [22–24] and indicate the necessity of developing methods to sort tooth bud cell populations and to generate populations that are enriched in epithelial and mesenchymal PNDSC. Once purified homogeneous DSC populations are generated, the molecular and cellular properties of these cells can be assessed more easily, providing a molecular profile that can be manipulated for tooth tissue engineering applications.

Furthermore, bioengineered tooth crowns forming as discrete, very small, although anatomically correct, structures indicate the need to devise strategies to guide the placement and interactions of epithelial and mesen-chymal dental progenitor cells on the supporting scaffold in order to generate full-sized bioengineered dental tissues of predetermined size and shape.

Another property of PNDSC revealed by these studies is their slow growth, indicating that it likely is necessary to devise methods to hasten the formation of bioengineered replacement teeth. If human progenitor tooth cells exhibit similar properties to lower mammals, such as pigs and rats, which is likely, it can be estimated that human PNDSC require approx-imately 1 year or longer to generate bioengineered human teeth based on the growth rates of naturally formed human teeth. Because a year is a long time to wait for replacement teeth to grow, it is advantageous to devise methods to hasten the formation of bioengineered teeth if this approach is to attain widespread clinical application.

Generating enriched dental progenitor cell populations

Based on the need to generate enriched, homogenous epithelial and mes-enchymal PNDSC populations for tooth tissue engineering applications, the authors use two approaches. The first is based on the ability to sort stem cells using antibodies that recognize the antigen, STRO-1, a carbohydrate moiety present on many types of stem cells [25,26]. Heterogeneous tooth bud cell populations can be incubated with magnetic beads to which anti–STRO-1 antibody is linked covalently. The cells that express STRO-1 become bound to the magnetic beads, whereas the STRO-1 negative non–stem cells are washed off. The STRO-1 expressing stem cell populations then are released from the magnetic beads, resulting in an enriched PNDSC popula-tion. Enriched epithelial and mesenchymal DSC populations are generated initially by dissecting the enamel organ (containing the epithelial DSC) away from the pulp organ (containing the mesenchymal DSC) of the starting tooth bud and then immunosorting the resulting epithelial and mesenchymal cell populations separately. This approach allows for determination and comparison of the characteristics of epithelial versus mesenchymal dental cell populations.

A second approach to generating enriched DSC populations is to perform Hoechst 33342 dye profiling, taking advantage of the ability of certain stem cells to exhibit the capacity to efflux the dye, whereas non–stem cells retain the dye [27]. After labeling, the cells are sorted by flow cytometry to generate enriched populations of Hoechst 33342 negative (stem) cells, termed side population (SP) cells, and Hoechst 33342 retaining (non–stem cell) popula-tions. Once sorted, clonal epithelial and mesenchymal SP and non-SP cells can be expanded in vitro and tested in pairwise fashion (it takes epithelial and mesenchymal DSC to generate teeth) for their ability to initiate and maintain a developmental program for tooth development. Molecular and cellular profiling of identified DSC clones will provide insight into the molecules that confer "stemness" onto DSC, providing a molecular map that can be manipulated to facilitate dental tissue bioengineering applications.

Examining dental cell-scaffold interactions

As discussed previously, the interactions of the scaffold with the PNDSC is of importance in guiding the size, shape, and differentiation of bioengineered dental tissues. Teeth are unique in that they are highly mineralized—enamel is the hardest substance in the body [28,29]. But teeth are organs, and early tooth development resembles that of soft tissue organs, such as the heart and liver, in that they are derived from the interactions of two cell types—epithelial and mesenchymal [30–33]. The size and shape of mature, highly mineralized teeth is determined early in development by the epithelial and mesenchymal interactions directing the morphology of the soft epithelial and mesenchymal tissues before any mineralization. Subsequent interactive signaling between the dental epithelium and mesenchyme results in dental tissue differentiation, including the induction of dentin-forming odontoblasts, enamel-secreting ameloblasts, and the placement of enamel knot signaling centers designating the locations of tooth cusps and tooth identity [34]. To master the task of generating bioengineered teeth of predetermined size and shape successfully, manipulating very early epithelial-mesenchymal cell interactions must be learned, to guide the eventual formation of the highly mineralized tooth tissues. Early dental cell and biodegradable scaffold interactions are key to this process.

The authors' initial tooth tissue engineering studies used biodegradable polyester scaffolds, fabricated from polyglycolic acid (or polyglycolide) (PGA) and polylactic acid (or polylactide) (PLA) [35]. The widespread use of these materials, alone and in combination with other materials, demonstrates their usefulness in bioengineering hard and soft tissues, including bone [36–38], skin [39] and intestine [15]. The authors' results suggest that the use of alternative scaffold materials or designs may facilitate the formation of bioengineered teeth of predetermined size and shape [20,40]. They are, therefore, investigating the use of alternative scaffold materials, including PGA/PLGA, collagen [41], silk [42], and combinations of these materials combined with modified scaffold designs. Recent progress in nanotechnology and 3-D imprinting–based scaffold fabrication and cell-seeding techniques [43] suggests the usefulness of these methods to guide the orientation and interactions of early dental epithelial and mesenchymal cell layers as they are seeded initially onto biodegradable scaffolds. In this way, the authors hope to guide the critical early dental cell proliferation and interactions that precede the morphologic events of tooth development, thereby defining the size and shape of teeth.

The authors also are working to define in vitro assays that can be used to screen for the early epithelial and mesenchymal dental cell interactions characterizing tooth initiation, including the use of hydrogel materials and technologies to facilitate in vitro characterizations of PNDSC [44,45]. The ability to screen clonal epithelial and mesenchymal PNDSC lines rapidly for pairwise combinations whose interactions result in tooth induction will facilitate the identification of appropriate cell lines for future character-izations in tooth tissue engineering applications.

Current research goals

The authors' current research efforts in whole tooth tissue engineering are focused on three areas: (1) molecular profiling of epithelial and mesenchy-mal PNDSC to define the genes whose coordinated expression confers on these cells the ability to adopt dental cell differentiation fates; (2) defining methods of manipulating PNDSC via cell-cell and cell-scaffold interactions to generate bioengineered tooth tissues of predetermined size and shape that exhibit similar physical and mechanical properties to those exhibited by nat-urally formed dental tissues; and (3) promoting the formation of bioengi-neered tooth root structures, including cementum, periodontal ligament, and alveolar bone. Progress in each of these areas that will facilitate whole tooth tissue engineering efforts is described briefly.

Molecular profiling of epithelial and mesenchymal dental stem cells

It is the authors' hope that molecular profiling of epithelial and mesen-chymal stem cells will provide important information. It is possible that the expression of certain growth factors, at discrete times and in discrete cell populations, may stimulate the initiation and maintenance of a tooth differentiation program that leads eventually to the formation of bioengi-neered dental tissues or even whole teeth. Once these gene profiles are deter-mined, it may be possible to manipulate these signaling cascades to modify tooth development programs for dental tissue engineering purposes. For ex-ample, it may be possible to hasten replacement tooth development by over-expressing certain genes or prolonging or delaying the expression of other genes. In addition, it may be possible to induce nonodontogenic progenitor stem cells to adopt a tooth differentiation fate by inducing in them the ex-pression of dental progenitor cell genes. An application for this is the ability to generate postnatal dental epithelial stem cell populations from alternative adult epithelial tissues. The absence of dental epithelial stem cells in adults is believed to be because once they form tooth crown enamel, they seem to lose their ability to self-renew and, instead, terminally differentiate to form tooth root tissues [46]. This phenomenon results in the absence of epithelial DSC populations in erupted teeth, precluding their use in tooth tissue engineering applications. It is possible that if the molecular profile of epithelial DSC can be determined (ie, if those genes can be identified whose combined

THE DENTAL
CLINICS
OF NORTH AMERICA

ELSEVIER
SAUNDERS

Dent Clin N Am 50 (2006) 205–216

The Engineering of Craniofacial Tissues in the Laboratory: A Review of Biomaterials for Scaffolds and Implant Coatings

Haru Abukawa, DDS, PhD[a],
Maria Papadaki, DMD, MD[a],
Mailikai Abulikemu, MD, MSc[a], Jeremy Leaf, BA[a],
Joseph P. Vacanti, MD[b],
Leonard B. Kaban, DMD, MD[a],
Maria J. Troulis, DDS, MSc[a],*

[a]Department of Oral and Maxillofacial Surgery, Massachusetts General Hospital,
Boston, MA, USA
[b]Department of Pediatric Surgery, Massachusetts General Hospital, Boston, MA, USA

A majority of craniomaxillofacial reconstructive procedures are performed to replace or construct missing or damaged skeletal structures. These operations require the harvesting of bone or soft tissue from distant donor sites. The donor site operation often results in greater morbidity than the primary reconstructive procedure and there may not be adequate quantities of bone available for harvesting in children. Furthermore, there is unpredictable loss of bone graft volume during the remodeling process.

Langer and Vacanti define tissue engineering as "an interdisciplinary field that applies the principles of engineering and the life sciences toward the development of biological substitutes that restore, maintain or improve tissue function" [1]. One tissue engineering strategy is based on harvesting

This work was funded in part by the Center for Integration of Medicine and Innovative Technology (CIMIT), Therics Corp, the Hanson Foundation, and the Massachusetts General Hospital Oral and Maxillofacial Surgery Education and Research Fund.

* Corresponding author. Department of Oral and Maxillofacial Surgery, Massachusetts General Hospital, Warren Building 1201, 55 Fruit Street, Boston, MA 02114.

E-mail address: mtroulis@partners.org (M.J. Troulis).

progenitor or stem cells, expanding and then, differentiating them into cells that have the potential to form new tissue (eg, bone) or organ (eg, tooth). The harvested cells are seeded on scaffolds. These scaffolds are fabricated in the laboratory to resemble the structure of the desired tissue or organ to be replaced. Much of the current tissue engineering research is directed toward the areas of cell manipulation (isolation, expansion, and differentiation) and scaffold design (biomaterials, design, and fabrication). This article reviews biomaterials available for use in craniomaxillofacial tissue (bone) engineering, coatings applied to scaffolds, and scaffold fabrication techniques.

Biomaterials for bone tissue engineering

The role of the scaffold in tissue engineering is to provide a matrix of a specific geometric configuration on which seeded cells may grow to produce the desired tissue or organ. The physical and chemical characteristics of a scaffold play a significant role in cell proliferation and tissue in-growth.

Biomaterials used as scaffolds for bone tissue engineering are classified into two broad categories: naturally derived and synthetic. Advantages of naturally derived scaffolds include the ability to support cellular invasion and proliferation. Synthetic materials offer ease of processing and mechanical strength [2].

Biomaterials used in tissue engineering also may be divided into ceramics and polymers [3]. These biomaterials may be produced in solid blocks, sheets, porous sponges or foams, or hydrogels. Historically, many of these substances have been used as bone substitutes, sutures, meshes, fixation devices, and dressings.

Bone is composed of an organic (polymer) component, primarily collagen, and a mineral (ceramic) component, primarily hydroxyapatite (HA) [4]. Currently, these individual components are being studied for use as scaffolds in tissue engineering. Novel biodegradable materials with improved mechanical properties, cell-interaction properties, and process ability also are being developed [5].

Scaffolds for use in bone tissue engineering must allow for: (1) easy cell penetration, distribution, and proliferation [6]; (2) permeability of the culture medium [7]; (3) in vivo vascularization (once implanted) [8,9]; (4) maintenance of osteoblastic cell phenotype; (5) adequate mechanical stiffness [10]; (6) proper biodegradation (rate and inflammatory response) and eventual total replacement by bone [11]; and (7) ease of fabrication (including 3-D printing). To date, the ideal scaffold that meets all these criteria has not been developed.

Biomaterials used as scaffolds: ceramics

Natural or synthetic HA and beta-tricalcium phosphate (β-TCP) are ceramics used in bone tissue engineering. Ceramic biomaterials structurally are similar to the inorganic component of bone. They are biocompatible, osteoconductive, and may bind directly to bone. They are protein- thus, stimulate no immunologic reaction [12]. Furthermore, ceram rials have long degradation times (many years) in vivo [3].

HA is a well-known biomaterial used for many decades as a bone substitute for small defects of the jaws. It may be derived from bovine bone (deproteinized) or coralline or made as a pure synthetic. It was one of the first biomaterials used as a scaffold, seeded with osteoprogenitor cells from periosteum or bone marrow, for bone and cartilage engineering [3,13]. Currently, investigators (primarily in Japan and Europe) continue to study HA for use as a scaffold in bone tissue engineering [14,15]. Major disadvantages of HA are that it is brittle, it has little mechanical strength, it does not resorb, and the pore size cannot be controlled easily by conventional processing methods [16].

Harris and Cooper assessed the osteogenic potential of bone marrow–derived human mesenchymal stem cells (hMSC) seeded on HA scaffolds [17]. The constructs (hMSC + HA scaffolds) were implanted into a dorsal pouch in the skin of mice for 5 weeks. Regardless of the type of HA scaffold used (coralline HA, bovine bone-derived HA, or synthetic HA/TCP), histomorphometric analysis revealed minimal bone formation. The most bone formation (only 13.8% of total surface area) was documented in the synthetic HA/TCP scaffolds [17]. In contrast to this study, Boo and colleagues show "active bone formation" when using a HA scaffold [18]. Others find a higher cell density on HA scaffolds when combined with TCP and fibrin [19].

TCP is a naturally occurring material comprising calcium and phosphorous and is used as a ceramic bone substitute in craniomaxillofacial and orthopedic surgery. This material has the advantage that it can be made into specifically shaped scaffolds by 3-D printing technology. Olsen and coworkers use β-TCP to fabricate 3-D printed scaffolds for in vitro bone engineering using porcine bone marrow progenitor cells. TCP scaffolds are shown to maintain their shape and allow for good cell penetration and bone formation in this in vitro model. The comparison of β-TCP scaffolds with PLGA (D,L-lactic-co-glycolic acid) scaffolds shows that similar cell penetration and bone formation occur with both materials [20].

Boo and colleagues compared β-TCP and HA as scaffolds for bone engineering. The scaffolds were seeded with MSC and implanted in subcutaneous sites. Histologic examination after 8 weeks revealed active bone formation in HA and TCP scaffolds [18].

TCP degrades either through osteoclastic resorption (phagocytosis) or by chemical dissolution by the interstitial fluid [21]. β-TCP is expected to degrade 3 times faster than HA; however, degradation in vivo remains controversial [22,23]. In vivo experiments using rabbits demonstrate that TCP may resorb and be replaced by newly formed bone within 3 months [24]. Handschel and coworkers, however, show that no TCP degradation occurred, even after 6 months, under nonloading conditions in a rat model. Generally, the predictability of ceramic degradation is poor [25]. Furthermore, the extent of degradation depends on many factors, such as crystallinity, porosity, density, form, size, the host, and implantation site [26]. Furthermore, HA and TCP are not strong enough scaffolds to provide mechanical strength when replacing load bearing skeletal structures.

Biomaterials used as scaffolds: polymers

The common polymers studied for craniomaxillofacial bone tissue engineering include synthetic polyesters, such as polyglycolic acid (PGA), polylactic acid (PLA) [27], and polycaplactone (PCL) [28]. Natural polymers, such as collagen and hyaluronic acid, alginate, and agarose, also are studied as scaffolds. Recently, copolymers of polyethylene oxide and polypropylene oxide, known as pluronics, have been developed in the form of injectable hydrogels [29].

Polymers seeded with chondrocytes were used to engineer a human ear, temporomandibular joint disc, and meniscal-shaped constructs [30–32]. Advantages of synthetic polymers include the ease and control of synthesis, their unlimited supply, and non–cell-mediated degradation. Biodegradable synthetic polymers can be formulated to possess desirable pore features and shape [33–35]. Disadvantages include lack of mechanical strength, difficulty in 3-D fabrication (specifically, 3-D printing), uncontrollable shrinkage, questionable cell-polymer interactions, and possible local toxicity resulting from acidic degradation products [35].

PGA has been used for many years as a resorbable suture (for example, Dexon [American Cyanamid, Pearl River, New York]). It is the first polymeric scaffold used to tissue engineer cartilage [3]. PGA is insoluble in water, and glycolic acid is the final product of degradation resulting local acidosis and potential tissue damage [35].

PLA is the polymer of lactic acid and is used as a scaffold. PLA is more hydrophobic than PGA and more resistant to hydrolysis. It is degradated into lactic acid, which also can be locally toxic to tissues [35].

PLGA is a copolymer of PGA and PLA. The suture material, Vicryl (Ethicon, Somerville, New Jersey), is composed of PLGA. Abukawa and coworkers used PLGA to make a 3-D scaffold in the shape of a porcine mandibular condyle (Fig. 1). The scaffold was seeded with porcine MSC in this autologous model. Bone formation occurred, however, only at the surface of the construct after 6 weeks of in vitro culture [36]. Abukawa and colleagues designed and fabricated a novel scaffold composed of PLGA with heterogenous pore sizes (small, 20-m to 200-m diameter, and large, 1-mm to 2-mm diameter), called the fused interconnected scaffold. MSC harvested from the ilium of a minipig were combined with these scaffolds. After only 10 days in a bioreactor, cultured constructs were implanted into mandibular defects of the same minipig and allowed to heal for 6 weeks. Histologic examination showed bone to bridge the defects (Fig. 2) [37]. The degradation rate or resultant local tissue effects were not studied, however. Furthermore, these scaffolds lacked strength and are not amenable to easy 3-D printing technology.

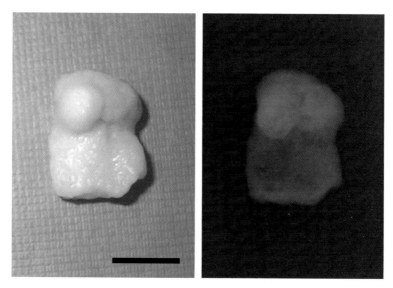

Fig. 1. Formation of a mandibular condyle in vitro by tissue engineering. Engineered construct consisting of bone and scafffold. Bar = 15 mm. (*From* Abukawa H, Terai H, Hannouche D, et al. Formation of a mandibular condyle in vitro by tissue engineering. J Oral Maxillofac Surg 2003;61:98; with permission.)

Currently available scaffold materials are less than ideal because of inadequate bone formation, lack of sufficient penetration of cells and bone throughout the scaffold, inadequate degradation properties, or inadequate mechanical stiffness.

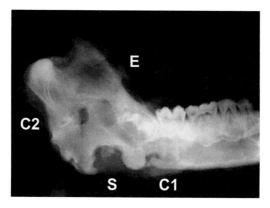

Fig. 2. Reconstruction of mandibular defects with autologous tissue-engineered bone. Reconstructed mandible with empty control (E), experimental contructs (C1 and C2), and control scaffold only (S). (*From* Abukawa H, Shin M, Williams WB, et al. Reconstruction of mandibular defects with autologous tissue-engineered bone. J Oral Maxillofac Surg 2004;62:604; with permission.)

New technologies for scaffold fabrication

New scaffold fabrication techniques are being developed, such as solid freeform fabrication (SFF). Products are designed on a computer screen as 3-D models with information from CT or MRI scans. Ideally, after implantation, a construct is organized into normal healthy tissue as the scaffold degrades. The goal of this technology is to fabricate a scaffold with accurate patient specific macrostructure (3-D shape) and microstructure (porosity and interconnected channels) for ideal nutrient flow and tissue and vascular in-growth.

This technology is relatively new and SFF machines for medical applications are available only at a few institutions, such as University of Michigan and Massachusetts Institute of Technology. Hollister's group uses this technology to tissue engineer bone with HA [38], PLA [39], and PCL [10]. Hollister's group finds this technology successful in producing bone in an immunocompromised mouse model [38]. Lin and coworkers also demonstrate that this method could produce highly porous structures that match human trabecular bone by introducing the homogenization-based topology optimization alogorithm [40]. Scheck and colleagues [40a] use genetically modified primary human gingival fibroblasts and HA scaffolds to produce bone. Williams and coworkers use PCL scaffolds and bone morphogenetic protein-7 (BMP-7)–induced human gingival fibroblasts cells to produce bone [10].

One SFF technique, the 3-D printing technology, is a manufacturing process that creates parts directly from a computer model used in the production of a complex 3-D scaffold. The parts are built by spreading a layer of powder repetitively and selectively joining the powder in the layer through the inkjet printing of a binder material [41]. Moreover, using multiple feeds, it becomes possible to manufacture scaffolds with various architectural qualities that can maintain multiple cell types on each layer, thus closely mimicking the anatomic features of a tissue or organ. Tissue engineering bone using this technique demonstrates ability of bone formation in vitro using porous PLGA/TCP composite scaffolds [42].

Lessons learned: implant coatings

The application of coatings to dental and orthopedic implants began approximately 20 years ago and has become a common practice in implant production [43]. The aim of coating implants was to increase biocompatibility and improve bone formation at the implant-bone interface.

HA is used more than any other coating to enhance osseointegration of titanium dental implants [44]. Several recent studies to measure the effect HA coatings have on titanium implants. One study followed 120 patients who received a total of 634 implants to assess the effect of implant coating (HA) on osseoointegration. Osseointegration was measured as a function of probing depth and micromobility. One year after implantation, results revealed a significantly smaller degree of micromobility in the HA-coated implants compared with noncoated ones [45]. This difference between the two groups declined steadily, and 3 years after implantation, the groups had no significant difference in micromobility. It was concluded that HA accelerated the initial rate of osseointegration.

Schwartz-Arad and colleagues compared marginal bone loss and 12-year survival rates of HA-coated implants to those of pure titanium implants. The average marginal bone loss was significantly higher ($P < .001$) among the HA-coated implants compared with the pure titanium implants, but the 12-year survival rates for the HA-coated implants were significantly higher than for those with the pure titanium implants [46].

Issues concerning the degradation of implant coatings have been raised, as it is believed that HA coatings tend to "peel" away and, because this product is not biodegradable, may cause implant failure [47].

One of the potential benefits of using implant coatings is that the materials can be used as a drug delivery system. This would be most useful in tissue engineering scaffolds. These may include growth factors and osteogenic supplements. In a recent experiment, recombinant human BMP-2 (rhBMP-2) was incorporated into the structure of calcium phosphate coatings used to coat titanium implants. The objective of this experiment was to combine these osteoinductive properties of rhBMP-2 with the osteoconductive properties of calcium phosphate coatings. It was found that the bioactive properties of rhBMP-2 were not affected by the process of being integrated with the HA [48].

In a similar experiment, hepatocyte growth factor (HGF) was incorporated into discs made of HA. HGF is a growth factor known to promote angiogenesis. This is a desirable property for implant coatings, because vascularization is an essential part of the bone formation. In this experiment, the effect of the HGF on osteoblast differentiation was observed in vitro. The results show that the HGF coatings induced alkaline phosphatase activity to a much greater extent than the plain HA coatings [49].

Recently, Wang and coworkers studied the prospect of using a mother-of-pearl coating on dental implants [47]. Previous studies found that nacre (mother of pearl) could stimulate bone cell differentiation and induce bone formation [50]. An advantage to nacre coatings is that the material is biodegradable, so it should not remain trapped at the implant/bone interface and interfere with long-term implant integration.

Smart scaffolds: the future

One of the basic roles of a scaffold in bone tissue engineering is to act as a carrier for cells and to maintain the space and create an environment in which the cells can proliferate and produce the desired bone matrix. Transplanted cells often lose the desired function upon transfer from the in vitro culture system to the in vivo recipient site [51,52]. To address these problems, scaffolds with the ability to deliver biochemical factors at a predetermined rate for a definitive time period are being developed [53]. These smart scaffolds have the advantage of being able to: (1) promote early capillary invasion [54], (2) maintain cell activity and desired phenotype [55], and (3) induce osteoblastic differentiation of existing progenitor cells in the recipient tissue [56,57].

Early reconstitution of the capillary system (ie, vascularization) is critical for tissue-engineered bone survival and function. Smith and colleagues report that sustained delivery of vascular endothelial growth factor enhances vascularization at the location of transplanted cells, which contributes to their survival [9]. The transplanted cells, therefore, subsequently proliferate and produce bone matrix at the reconstruction site.

Adult stem cells can be differentiated into osteoblasts when triggered by osteogenic supplements (100 nM dexamethasone, 50 µg/mL ascorbic acid, and 10 mM beta-glycerophosphate) [58,59]. Based on this data, Kim and colleagues designed a biodegradable poly (PLGA) scaffold that releases osteogenic media (containing dexamethasone and ascorbic acid) in vitro and in vivo [55,60]. Similarly, Zhang and coworkers used an ascorbic acid-containing polymer scaffold (lysine-di-isocyanate [LDI]-glycerol-polyethylene glycol [PEG]-ascorbic acid [AA]) that supports osteoblast proliferation and bone formation [61].

BMP are shown to initiate osteogenic differentiation in stem cells [62,63]. Furthermore, BMP have the unique ability to induce de novo bone and cartilage formation when implanted at ectopic sites [56,57]. A PLGA scaffold system capable of sustained BMP-4 is combined with bone marrow cells and reported to promote bone formation [54,64].

Bone tissue development is a highly coordinated process that involves various biologic factors. The ability to deliver multiple growth factors to a recipient site also may be a promising strategy to enhance bone formation, and the combination BMP-4 and vascular endothelial growth factor released from PLGA scaffolds is reported to enhance bone formation [54,64].

Release kinetics in drug delivery systems are predictable in vitro. In vivo, however, the environment is more complex, making it more difficult to predict the material degradation process. Therefore, maintaining drug release within the therapeutic range is one of the keys of an effective drug delivery system for tissue engineering bone in vivo. In fact, degradation products of polymers create an acidic environment in vivo [65,66]. An acidic environment associated with biodegradation increases the release of rhBMP-2 from the PLGA/calcium-phosphate cement composite in vitro compared with PLGA [67]. Zhang and colleagues demonstrate that the degradation products of LDI-glycerol-AA polymer do not affect the pH [68]. For effective controlled release, further experiments using biodegradable materials should be performed to optimize drug delivery system, for bone tissue engineering.

These "smart" materials may revolutionize tissue-engineering research, because controlled release of biochemical and growth factors from a scaffold may enhance cell penetration, proliferation, differentiation, and bone matrix production and improve vascularization of grafts.

Acknowledgments

The authors thank Mr. Brad Oriel of Bates College for critically reading the manuscript.

References

[1] Langer R, Vacanti JP. Tissue engineering. Science 1993;260:920–6.
[2] Rosso F, Marino G, Giordano A, et al. Smart materials as scaffolds for tissue engineering. J Cell Physiol 2005;203:465–70.
[3] Vacanti CA, Bonassar LJ. An overview of tissue engineered bone. Clin Orthop Relat Res 1999;367(Suppl):S375–81.
[4] Sachlos E, Reis N, Ainsley C, et al. Novel collagen scaffolds with predefined internal morphology made by solid freeform fabrication. Biomaterials 2003;24:1487–97.
[5] Muschler GF, Nakamoto C, Griffith LG. Engineering principles of clinical cell-based tissue engineering. J Bone Joint Surg Am 2004;86-A:1541–58.
[6] Crane GM, Ishaug SL, Mikos AG. Bone tissue engineering. Nat Med 1995;1:1322–4.
[7] Glowacki J. Engineered cartilage, bone, joints, and menisci. Potential for temporomandibular joint reconstruction. Cells Tissues Organs 2001;169:302–8.
[8] Frerich B, Lindemann N, Kurtz-Hoffmann J, et al. In vitro model of a vascular stroma for the engineering of vascularized tissues. Int J Oral Maxillofac Surg 2001;30:414–20.
[9] Smith MK, Peters MC, Richardson TP, et al. Locally enhanced angiogenesis promotes transplanted cell survival. Tissue Eng 2004;10:63–71.
[10] Williams JM, Adewunmi A, Schek RM, et al. Bone tissue engineering using polycaprolactone scaffolds fabricated via selective laser sintering. Biomaterials 2005;26:4817–27.
[11] El-Ghannam AR. Advanced bioceramic composite for bone tissue engineering: design principles and structure-bioactivity relationship. J Biomed Mater Res A 2004;69:490–501.
[12] Burg KJ, Porter S, Kellam JF. Biomaterial developments for bone tissue engineering. Biomaterials 2000;21:2347–59.
[13] Ohgushi H, Caplan AI. Stem cell technology and bioceramics: from cell to gene engineering. J Biomed Mater Res 1999;48:913–27.
[14] Fischer EM, Layrolle P, Van Blitterswijk CA, et al. Bone formation by mesenchymal progenitor cells cultured on dense and microporous hydroxyapatite particles. Tissue Eng 2003;9: 1179–88.
[15] Kokubo T, Kim HM, Kawashita M. Novel bioactive materials with different mechanical properties. Biomaterials 2003;24:2161–75.
[16] Chu TM, Orton DG, Hollister SJ, et al. Mechanical and in vivo performance of hydroxyapatite implants with controlled architectures. Biomaterials 2002;23:1283–93.
[17] Harris CT, Cooper LF. Comparison of bone graft matrices for human mesenchymal stem cell-directed osteogenesis. J Biomed Mater Res A 2004;68:747–55.
[18] Boo JS, Yamada Y, Okazaki Y, et al. Tissue-engineered bone using mesenchymal stem cells and a biodegradable scaffold. J Craniofac Surg 2002;13:231–9 [discussion: 40–3].
[19] Phang MY, Ng MH, Tan KK, et al. Evaluation of suitable biodegradable scaffolds for engineered bone tissue. Med J Malaysia 2004;59(Suppl B):198–9.
[20] Olson DP, Abukawa H, Vacanti JP, et al., Three-dimensional printed beta-TCP scaffold for bone tissue engineering [abstract]. Presented at the American Association of Oral &

Maxillofacial Surgeons 2004 Annual Meeting. San Francisco (CA), September 29–October 2, 2004.

[21] Zerbo IR, Bronckers AL, de Lange G, et al. Localisation of osteogenic and osteoclastic cells in porous beta-tricalcium phosphate particles used for human maxillary sinus floor elevation. Biomaterials 2005;26:1445–51.

[22] Koerten HK, van der Meulen J. Degradation of calcium phosphate ceramics. J Biomed Mater Res 1999;44:78–86.

[23] Handschel J, Wiesmann HP, Stratmann U, et al. TCP is hardly resorbed and not osteoconductive in a non-loading calvarial model. Biomaterials 2002;23:1689–95.

[24] Bhaskar SN, Brady JM, Getter L, et al. Biodegradable ceramic implants in bone. Electron and light microscopic analysis. Oral Surg Oral Med Oral Pathol 1971;32:336–46.

[25] Gosain AK, Persing JA. Biomaterials in the face: benefits and risks. J Craniofac Surg 1999; 10:404–14.

[26] Theiss F, Apelt D, Brand B, et al. Biocompatibility and resorption of a brushite calcium phosphate cement. Biomaterials 2005;26:4383–94.

[27] Isogai N, Landis W, Kim TH, et al. Formation of phalanges and small joints by tissue-engineering. J Bone Joint Surg [Am] 1999;81:306–16.

[28] Yoshimoto H, Shin YM, Terai H, et al. A biodegradable nanofiber scaffold by electrospinning and its potential for bone tissue engineering. Biomaterials 2003;24:2077–82.

[29] Xu XL, Lou J, Tang T, et al. Evaluation of different scaffolds for BMP-2 genetic orthopedic tissue engineering. J Biomed Mater Res B Appl Biomater 2005;75(2):289–303.

[30] Cao Y, Vacanti JP, Paige KT, et al. Transplantation of chondrocytes utilizing a polymer-cell construct to produce tissue-engineered cartilage in the shape of a human ear. Plast Reconstr Surg 1997;100:297–302 [discussion: 3–4].

[31] Puelacher WC, Vacanti JP, Ferraro NF, et al. Femoral shaft reconstruction using tissue-engineered growth of bone. Int J Oral Maxillofac Surg 1996;25:223–8.

[32] Weng Y, Cao Y, Silva CA, et al. Tissue-engineered composites of bone and cartilage for mandible condylar reconstruction. J Oral Maxillofac Surg 2001;59:185–90.

[33] Behravesh E, Yasko AW, Engel PS, et al. Synthetic biodegradable polymers for orthopaedic applications. Clin Orthop Relat Res 1999;367(Suppl):S118–29.

[34] Lendlein A, Langer R. Biodegradable, elastic shape-memory polymers for potential biomedical applications. Science 2002;296:1673–6.

[35] Gunatillake PA, Adhikari R. Biodegradable synthetic polymers for tissue engineering. Eur Cell Mater 2003;5:1–16 [discussion].

[36] Abukawa H, Terai H, Vacanti JP, et al. Reconstruction of a mandible condyle by tissue engineering. J Oral Maxillofac Surg 2003;61:94–100.

[37] Abukawa H, Shin M, Williams WB, et al. Reconstruction of mandibular defects with autologous tissue-engineered bone. J Oral Maxillofac Surg 2004;62:601–6.

[38] Schek RM, Taboas JM, Segvich SJ, et al. Engineered osteochondral grafts using biphasic composite solid free-form fabricated scaffolds. Tissue Eng 2004;10:1376–85.

[39] Taboas JM, Maddox RD, Krebsbach PH, et al. Indirect solid free form fabrication of local and global porous, biomimetic and composite 3D polymer-ceramic scaffolds. Biomaterials 2003;24:181–94.

[40] Lin CY, Kikuchi N, Hollister SJ. A novel method for biomaterial scaffold internal architecture design to match bone elastic properties with desired porosity. J Biomech 2004;37:623–36.

[40a] Scheck RM, Wilke FN, Hollister SJ, et al. Combined use of designed scaffolds and adenoviral gene therapy for skeletal tissue engineering. Biomaterials 2006;27:1160–6.

[41] Curodeau A, Sachs E, Caldarise S. Design and fabrication of cast orthopedic implants with freeform surface textures from 3-D printed ceramic shell. J Biomed Mater Res 2000;53:525–35.

[42] Sherwood JK, Riley SL, Palazzolo R, et al. A three-dimensional osteochondral composite scaffold for articular cartilage repair. Biomaterials 2002;23:4739–51.

[43] Sun L, Berndt CC, Gross KA, et al. Material fundamentals and clinical performance of plasma-sprayed hydroxyapatite coatings: a review. J Biomed Mater Res 2001;58:570–92.

[44] Baltag I, Watanabe K, Kusakari H, Taguchi N, et al. Long-term changes of hydroxyapatite-coated dental implants. J Biomed Mater Res 2000;53:76–85.

[45] Geurs NC, Jeffcoat RL, McGlumphy EA, et al. Influence of implant geometry and surface characteristics on progressive osseointegration. Int J Oral Maxillofac Implants 2002;17: 811–5.

[46] Schwartz-Arad D, Mardinger O, Levin L, et al. Marginal bone loss pattern around hydroxy-apatite-coated versus commercially pure titanium implants after up to 12 years of follow-up. Int J Oral Maxillofac Implants 2005;20:238–44.

[47] Wang XX, Xie L, Wang R. Biological fabrication of nacreous coating on titanium dental implant. Biomaterials 2005;26:6229–32.

[48] Liu Y, Hunziker EB, Layrolle P, et al. Bone morphogenetic protein 2 incorporated into biomimetic coatings retains its biological activity. Tissue Eng 2004;10:101–8.

[49] Hossain M, Irwin R, Baumann MJ, et al. Hepatocyte growth factor (HGF) adsorption kinetics and enhancement of osteoblast differentiation on hydroxyapatite surfaces. Biomaterials 2005;26:2595–602.

[50] Atlan G, Delattre O, Berland S, et al. Interface between bone and nacre implants in sheep. Biomaterials 1999;20:1017–22.

[51] Gundle R, Joyner CJ, Triffitt JT. Human bone tissue formation in diffusion chamber culture in vivo by bone-derived cells and marrow stromal fibroblastic cells. Bone 1995;16:597–601.

[52] Haynesworth SE, Goshima J, Goldberg VM, et al. Characterization of cells with osteogenic potential from human marrow. Bone 1992;13:81–8.

[53] Langer R. Implantable controlled release systems. Pharmacol Ther 1983;21:35–51.

[54] Huang YC, Kaigler D, Rice KG, et al. Combined angiogenic and osteogenic factor delivery enhances bone marrow stromal cell-driven bone regeneration. J Bone Miner Res 2005;20: 848–57.

[55] Kim H, Suh H, Jo SA, et al. In vivo bone formation by human marrow stromal cells in biodegradable scaffolds that release dexamethasone and ascorbate-2-phosphate. Biochem Biophys Res Commun 2005;332:1053–60.

[56] Sampath TK, Muthukumaran N, Reddi AH. Isolation of osteogenin, an extracellular matrix-associated, bone-inductive protein, by heparin affinity chromatography. Proc Natl Acad Sci U S A 1987;84:7109–13.

[57] Wozney JM, Rosen V, Celeste AJ, et al. Novel regulators of bone formation: molecular clones and activities. Science 1988;242:1528–34.

[58] Pittenger MF, Mackay AM, Beck SC, et al. Multilineage potential of adult human mesenchymal stem cells. Science 1999;284:143–7.

[59] Jaiswal N, Haynesworth SE, Caplan AI, et al. Osteogenic differentiation of purified, culture-expanded human mesenchymal stem cells in vitro. J Cell Biochem 1997;64:295–312.

[60] Kim H, Kim HW, Suh H. Sustained release of ascorbate-2-phosphate and dexamethasone from porous PLGA scaffolds for bone tissue engineering using mesenchymal stem cells. Biomaterials 2003;24:4671–9.

[61] Zhang JY, Doll BA, Beckman EJ, et al. Three-dimensional biocompatible ascorbic acid-containing scaffold for bone tissue engineering. Tissue Eng 2003;9:1143–57.

[62] Gori F, Thomas T, Hicok KC, et al. Differentiation of human marrow stromal precursor cells: bone morphogenetic protein-2 increases OSF2/CBFA1, enhances osteoblast commitment, and inhibits late adipocyte maturation. J Bone Miner Res 1999;14:1522–35.

[63] Hanada K, Dennis JE, Caplan AI. Stimulatory effects of basic fibroblast growth factor and bone morphogenetic protein-2 on osteogenic differentiation of rat bone marrow-derived mesenchymal stem cells. J Bone Miner Res 1997;12:1606–14.

[64] Simmons CA, Alsberg E, Hsiong S, et al. Dual growth factor delivery and controlled scaffold degradation enhance in vivo bone formation by transplanted bone marrow stromal cells. Bone 2004;35:562–9.

[65] Athanasiou KA, Niederauer GG, Agrawal CM. Sterilization, toxicity, biocompatibility and clinical applications of polylactic acid/polyglycolic acid copolymers. Biomaterials 1996;17: 93–102.

[66] Penco M, Marcioni S, Ferruti P, et al. Degradation behaviour of block copolymers containing poly(lactic-glycolic acid) and poly(ethylene glycol) segments. Biomaterials 1996;17: 1583–90.

[67] Ruhe PQ, Hedberg EL, Padron NT, et al. rhBMP-2 release from injectable poly(DL-lactic-co-glycolic acid)/calcium-phosphate cement composites. J Bone Joint Surg [Am] 2003; 85–A(Suppl 3):75–81.

[68] Zhang J, Doll BA, Beckman EJ, et al. A biodegradable polyurethane-ascorbic acid scaffold for bone tissue engineering. J Biomed Mater Res A 2003;67:389–400.

ELSEVIER
SAUNDERS

THE DENTAL
CLINICS
OF NORTH AMERICA

Dent Clin N Am 50 (2006) 217–228

Use of Growth Factors to Modify Osteoinductivity of Demineralized Bone Allografts: Lessons for Tissue Engineering of Bone

Barbara D. Boyan, PhD[a,*], Don M. Ranly, DDS, PhD[a],
Zvi Schwartz, DMD, PhD[a,b]

[a]Georgia Institute of Technology, Atlanta, GA, USA
[b]Hebrew University, Hadassah Faculty of Dental Medicine, Jerusalem, Israel

Bone grafting materials are used in oral and craniofacial surgery for a variety of applications. Where there is sufficient vascular supply and the amount of bone needed is small, clinicians often can use autologous bone harvested from the surgical site itself. Many different kinds of osteoconductive materials can be used effectively to augment the autologous bone, thereby providing needed structural support at the site. Materials of this kind include calcium phosphate ceramic particles, various forms of bioactive glass, and anorganic bone. Although these materials do not possess inherent osteogenic properties, they are biocompatible and provide surfaces that enable the migration of mesenchymal cells to the site where they differentiate into bone-forming cells and produce new bone.

For some patients, the supply of autologous bone is limited and harvesting bone from extraoral sites has its own morbidity. This is true particularly for older individuals, whose quality of bone stock may be compromised by osteoporosis or other conditions, including diabetes and renal failure. In these cases, it is advantageous to use alternative bone graft materials that are osteoconductive and osteogenic. Osteogenic materials are those that cause bone to form in an orthotopic site to a greater extent than is predicted

This work was supported by grants and gifts from Biora AB, BioMimetic Pharmaceuticals, the Musculoskeletal Transplant Foundation, DePuy Germany, LifeNet, Inc., the Genetics Institute, the Price Gilbert, Jr., Foundation, and the Georgia Research Alliance.

* Corresponding author. Institute for Bioengineering and Bioscience, 315 Ferst Drive NW, Atlanta, GA 30332-0363.

E-mail address: barbara.boyan@bme.gatech.edu (B.D. Boyan).

if the material were acting only as a substrate for cell migration and growth. They include bone marrow stromal cells, mesenchymal stem cells, and several growth factors shown to increase mesenchymal cell numbers or enhance osteoblastic differentiation (Box 1).

Osteoinductive materials are those that cause bone to form in sites that otherwise would not support bone formation (eg, muscle or fascia). When implanted in bone, osteoinductive agents recruit undifferentiated mesenchymal cells and induce their differentiation into cells required for bone formation, in particular chondrocytes and osteoblasts. These agents also act directly on osteoprogenitor cells and committed osteoblasts. When implanted in nonorthotopic sites, osteoinductive materials initiate the process of endochondral ossification in a manner similar to embryonic bone formation. Mesenchymal cells attracted to the implant differentiate into

---

Box 1. Bone graft products used for bone tissue engineering

Osteoinductive
Demineralized freeze-dried bone allograft (DFDBA)
Partially pure proteins (BMP)
BMP-2
BMP-4
BMP-7
BMP-9

Osteoconductive
Freeze-dried bone
Autograft
Ceramics
Bioglasses
Coral-derived
Deproteinized bovine bone
Polylactic acid (PLA)/polyglycolic acid (PGA)

Osteogenic
Mesenchymal stem cells (MSC)
Marrow
Platelet-rich plasma (PRP)
PRP + white blood cells (WBC)
Emdogain
Gene therapy
Fibroblast growth factor (FGF)
Peptide TP508
Peptide P15
Platelet-derived growth factor (PDGF)

chondrocytes, producing and calcifying cartilage matrix. Once this occurs, the calcified cartilage is invaded by blood vessels bringing osteoprogenitor cells. Bone is formed on the calcified cartilage scaffold, which is replaced by bone marrow, resulting in formation of a complete ossicle consisting of hematopoietic marrow surrounded by cortical bone [1].

The canonical osteoinductive material is demineralized bone, first described by Urist in 1965 [2]. At least part of the reason for the osteoinductivity of demineralized bone is the presence and release of osteoinductive proteins collectively known as BMP. Two of these proteins, BMP-2 and BMP-7 (osteogenic protein-1 [OP-1]), have been developed commercially for use as bone inductive materials. Both proteins initiate endochondral bone formation when implanted heterotopically [3,4] and stimulate bone formation clinically [5–7].

Although BMP are the most effective osteoinductive materials known, there are problems associated with their use. BMP are produced by bone cells and stored in the extracellular matrix of bone at low levels and always in the presence of one or more inhibitors [8,9]. This ensures that they are available when needed and that they are active only under specific conditions. When activated, the clearance rate for BMP is rapid. Thus, it is necessary to implant large concentrations of these proteins to have active protein present at the time when an appropriate responding cell population also is present. Moreover, BMPs are most effective when used with a carrier to retain the proteins at the implant site and to provide an osteoconductive matrix.

Other factors contribute to bone formation in a variety of ways. Given the ease of using osteoinductive demineralized bone as a bone graft substitute, it is of interest to find additives that can enhance its osteoinductivity. This article describes factors commonly used in dentistry and shows how these agents affect the osteoinduction ability of demineralized bone.

Methods and materials

Human demineralized freeze-dried bone allograft (DFDBA) was a gift from LifeNet (Virginia Beach, Virginia) and was provided in the form used clinically. DFDBA from 27 different donors was assayed for ability to induce new bone formation when implanted in gastrocnemius muscle of immunocompromised mice [10]. Batches that had high osteoinductivity or low osteoinductivity were selected for the studies (discussed later). The DFDBA was weighed (10 mg/implant), placed in gelatin capsules, and sterilized overnight under UV light. Immediately before implantation, the DFDBA was mixed with the agent of interest.

Recombinant human BMP-2 was supplied in saline (Genetics Institute; now Wyeth, Andover, Massachusetts) and used at a concentration of 100 ng/implant [11]. Emdogain (Biora AG, Malmo, Sweden; now Institut Straumann AB, Basel, Switzerland) was supplied as a powder and used at a concentration of 4 mg/implant [12]. Recombinant platelet-derived growth factor (PDGF)-BB (BioMimetics, Franklin, Tennessee) was supplied as a powder, dissolved in saline, and used at a concentration of 10 µg/implant [13]. PRP was prepared with the harvest machine [14] using blood from a healthy male subject. Each implant was mixed with 25-µL–activated PRP [15]. Activation of the PRP resulted in a 15-fold increase in total transforming growth factor-beta 1 (TGF-β1). Bio-Oss was extracted with 4 M guanidine hydrochloride and the extract was shown to contain low levels of BMP-2 and TGF-β1, among other proteins [12]. The proteins in the extract were concentrated, dialyzed against saline, and suspended in saline before mixing with DFDBA.

Materials were implanted bilaterally in the hind limb calf muscle of male Nu/Nu mice. These mice have a compromised immune system and, as a result, xenografts do not elicit an immune response. Tissues were examined for the presence of bone at 35 days (BMP-2, Emdogain, PDGF, or PRP) or 56 days (Bio-Oss) post implantation using histology and histomorphometry. The ability of the material to induce new bone formation was determined using a semiquantitative scoring system on paraffin sections stained with hematoxylin and eosin. If no material was found in the implanted tissue, the score was 0. If only the original implant was present, the score was 1. If new bone was present, the score was 2. If two or more ossicles were present, the score was 3; and if the new bone covered more than 70% of the section (magnification ×10), the score was 4. In addition, each section was analyzed by histomorphometric measurement of the area of new bone and the area of residual implant material.

For these experiments, each implant type was assessed using 8 individual implants, 2 identical implants per animal, 1 per leg. Data were analyzed by analysis of variance, and significant differences determined using the Bonferroni modification of the Student t test. Because these experiments were conducted at different times, to facilitate comparison of the results, treatment-to-control ratios were compared. In each case, the control was DFDBA alone and the treatment was DFDBA plus the agent. Studies using Bio-Oss are presented using actual values.

Results and discussion

Effects on osteoinduction

The ability of DFDBA to induce new bone formation varied with the additive used (Fig. 1). Addition of BMP-2 increased osteoinduction by almost 50% based on the bone induction score. DFDBA contains BMP-2, but the amount seems to vary among individuals [16]. Moreover, the formatting of BMP-2 within DFDBA is different from that of BMP-2 adsorbed to the surface of the graft particles. Studies suggest that the DFDBA particles must be resorbed for the BMP contained within the matrix to be released. DFDBA becomes, in effect, a time-release carrier for these factors. Surface-adsorbed BMP-2 is released in a burst and, as a result, has its greatest effects on cells

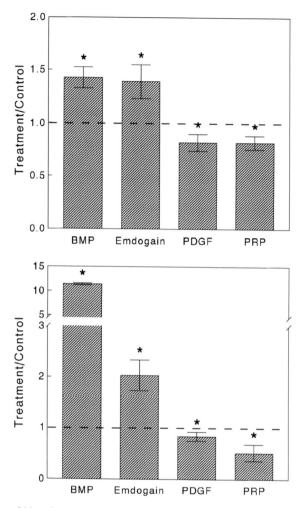

Fig. 1. Effects of bioactive agents on DFDBA-induced bone formation in the gastrocnemius muscle of immunocompromised mice. Nude mice were implanted bilaterally with human DFDBA plus recombinant human BMP-2, Emdogain, recombinant human PDGF-BB, or human PRP. The osteoinduction score was determined using a semiquantitative scale (*top panel*). The area of new bone was determined histomorphometrically (*bottom panel*). Data are treatment-to-control ratios for 8 implants. Values are expressed as means ± SEM. *, $P<0.05$ versus a treatment-to-control ratio of 1.

present at the implant site. Thus, the two forms of the morphogen work on distinctly different cell populations, and the combined effect is additive, if not synergistic. Other factors present in DFDBA also may contribute to the overall tissue response.

Emdogain had the same effect as BMP-2 on the osteoinduction score (see Fig. 1). This was an unexpected result. Emdogain is composed primarily of amelogenin and other proteins present in embryonic porcine tooth germs

[17]. It is reported to contain neither detectable BMP nor TGF-β [18]. Emdogain is believed to function as a matrix, potentially enhancing the recruitment and differentiation of mesenchymal cells [19]. It is possible that a trace component of Emdogain possesses osteoinductive properties. During embryonic development, the interaction of epithelial and mesenchymal tissues is critical for tissue morphogenesis. One or more of the factors that control this process may be present in Emdogain. Amelogenin itself seems important for coupling enamel formation via ectodermal ameloblasts and dentin formation via mesodermal odontoblasts [17]. More recently, amelogenin is shown to act on cells via growth factor–like signaling pathways [20]. Thus, Emdogain may act through similar mechanisms as DFDBA, resulting in an enhancement of DFDBA's osteoinductive properties.

In contrast to the increase in osteoinduction seen when DFDBA is implanted with BMP-2 or Emdogain, PDGF and PRP reduced osteoinductivity by approximately 20% (see Fig. 1). PDGF-BB is produced by platelets and is released by them at sites of injury. Unlike the morphogen, BMP-2, PDGF-BB is a growth factor, and its main effect is to stimulate DNA synthesis and cell proliferation [21]. Thus, in the presence of PDGF-BB, the number of mesenchymal cells, but not necessarily differentiated cells, is increased. If the differentiation stimulus provided by DFDBA is not great enough, then it is possible that the proliferative effect of the growth factor overwhelms the tissue response. The inhibitory effect of PDGF-BB on DFDBA-induced bone formation is concentration dependent and, at high concentrations, causes the chondrogenic phase of endochondral bone formation to persist [22]. At low concentrations, PDGF-BB does not inhibit DFDBA activity and, in an orthotopic site where other osteogenic signals are present, its effect on mesenchymal cell proliferation may result in increased bone formation. Clinical studies suggest that this is the case [23].

PDGF is a major component of PRP but not the only component. TGF-β also is enriched in PRP and, like PDGF, stimulates mesenchymal cell proliferation [24]. At high concentrations, TGF-β1 blocks terminal differentiation of growth plate chondrocytes and osteoblasts [25,26]. Whether or not this is a factor in the inhibition of bone formation via DFDBA is not known. PRP is used in dental surgery based on the hypothesis that it is an enrichment of autologous growth factors involved in wound healing. Many publications indicate that it improves bone healing in oral surgical applications. Part of this effect may be that PRP improves the handling properties of DFDBA. There is an increasing body of literature, however, that supports the authors' observation that PRP is inhibitory [27–30].

Effects on bone formation are specific to the factor used

The osteoinduction score indicates whether or not bone formation has occurred and gives some idea of the robustness of the effect, but it does not provide information about the quality of the osteoinduction. As shown in Fig. 1, BMP-2 had a much greater stimulatory effect on bone formation than Emdogain, even though both additives resulted in a comparable osteoinduction score. This can be attributed to the mechanisms involved. BMP-2 upregulates expression of transcription factors, such as RUNX-2, that regulate osteoblast phenotypic expression [31]. Thus, there are more bone cells and more bone. The lack of BMP in Emdogain suggests that its ability to enhance the osteoinductivity of DFDBA is the result of its properties as a bioactive matrix.

PDGF reduces new bone formation by DFDBA to a much lesser extent than PRP (see Fig. 1), suggesting that other components of PRP also are involved. TGF-β1 is one of these factors. PDGF and TGF-β1, however, can act directly on committed osteoblasts as autocrine and paracrine regulators of osteoblastic activity [24]. Although TGF-β1 is shown to block terminal differentiation [26], it does stimulate early states of osteoblastic maturation, including increased alkaline phosphatase activity. This supports the hypothesis that the environment is critical and that growth factors and cytokines present in an orthotopic site may be as important as those that are implanted.

Role of resorption rate in bone tissue engineering

Factors used to augment DFDBA also affect the rate of resorption of the implant material (Fig. 2). BMP-2 results in greater resorption of DFDBA than is seen when the allograft is implanted alone. This effect of BMP-2 is noted with other carriers, including polylactic acid/polyglycolic acid copolymer scaffolds implanted in nude mouse muscle [32] and when used clinically with bone graft [33]. One reason for this may be that BMP-2 activates resorbing cells in general; another may be that it stimulates the entire remodeling cycle and the graft or carrier material is resorbed as a byproduct of the osteoclastic resorption of bone [34]. For the most part, the net increase in bone formation overcomes any initial loss of carrier. In sites where retention of a carrier or bone graft substitute for longer periods of time is desirable, BMP-2 may not be the best approach overall.

Other additives, such as PDGF, are neutral with respect to DFDBA resorption (see Fig. 2). Even though PDGF was inhibitory with respect to bone formation, it was not because it stimulated bone resorption, supporting the interpretation of results (discussed previously). Emdogain and PRP delayed the rate at which DFDBA was resorbed, suggesting that factors present in these two complex agents might modulate bone remodeling in addition to bone formation. These are two different and complex mixtures that had distinctly different effects on DFDBA-induced osteogenesis, but it is likely that some factors are in common.

The case of Bio-Oss

Many of the approaches used to improve the predictability of DFDB-induced bone formation, such as those described previously, also are used

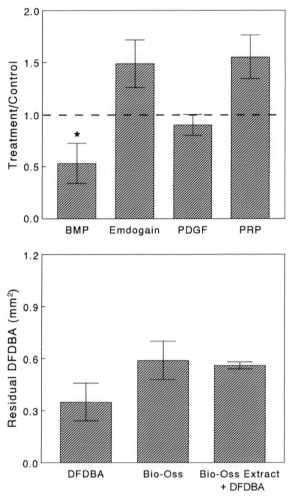

Fig. 2. Effects of bioactive agents on residual implant after DFDBA-induced bone formation in the gastrocnemius muscle of immunocompromised mice. At harvest, implanted tissues were examined for the presence of residual implant materials and the area measured. The top panel compares the effects of BMP-2, Emdogain, PDGF-BB, and PRP as treatment-to-control ratios. The bottom panel compares the amount of residual Bio-Oss to low-activity DFDBA with and without concentrated Bio-Oss extracts containing BMP-2 and TGF-β1. Data are means $\pm$ SEM for 8 implants of each kind.

with osteoconductive bone graft substitutes. The design of many of these materials is based on the chemical and physical structure of bone. The mineral phase of bone is a carbonate-substituted apatite and the crystallites are organized in a complex organic matrix. Various manufacturers have focused on the calcium phosphate chemistry and many of the new bone graft substitutes are fabricated to be resorbable within a reasonable time frame. The goal is for a material to be removed as new bone is formed, but this cannot always be achieved with ceramic materials of this kind.

An alternative approach is to produce materials that have the physical structure of bone mineral but with the organic matrix removed. The most common method used for this is to essentially incinerate the organic matrix, resulting in a sintered mineral phase that has the physical properties of calcified bone. Early studies indicate that although lower temperatures could remove most of the organic components of bone and retain bone mineral–like crystal structure, protein is protected by the mineral phase and could persist [35]. This is the case with Bio-Oss, which essentially is anorganic bovine bone, albeit with low levels of bioactive protein present, including BMP-2 [12]. As shown in Fig. 3, Bio-Oss by itself is not osteoinductive. After 56 days of implantation in nude mouse muscle, only the implant remained. When concentrated extracts of Bio-Oss proteins were added to low-activity DFDBA, however, osteoinduction ability of the composite implant was comparable to that seen typically in high-activity DFDBA. This is because of a twofold increase in new bone formation (see Fig. 3), similar to that seen with Emdogain. The Bio-Oss extracts were added to low-activity DFDBA [12], whereas Emdogain was added to high-activity DFDBA [36]. Thus, the effect of the Bio-Oss extract likely was the result of the added BMP-2. Despite this, the amount of DFDBA remaining at the implant site was unchanged (see Fig. 2). In an orthotopic site, a material, such as Bio-Oss, may be advantageous not only for its structural properties but also for the potential stimulus of inherent factors that stimulate bone formation.

Summary

Bone is a highly vascularized tissue and, under normal circumstances, even large defects heal with bone because of the local supply of mesenchymal stem cells within the bone marrow environment and the presence of osteoinductive agents within the bone matrix. In addition, factors released at the wound site or present within the hematoma enhance osteogenesis by recruiting progenitor cells and stimulating their proliferation and differentiation. When this process becomes dysregulated, either because of the size of the defect or because of other host-dependent factors, some form of bone tissue engineering may be necessary. Addition of multipotent autologous cells, such as those in bone marrow, and the addition of autologous bone as a structural element provide the optimal therapeutic approach. Often one or both of these are in limited supply and alternative approaches are needed. The lessons learned from the authors' study of DFDBA-induced bone formation illustrate those features of osteogenesis that may confound the use of tissue engineering strategies.

- The behavior of material may be different orthotopically and heterotopically. Factors that promote osteoinduction in muscle likely are effective

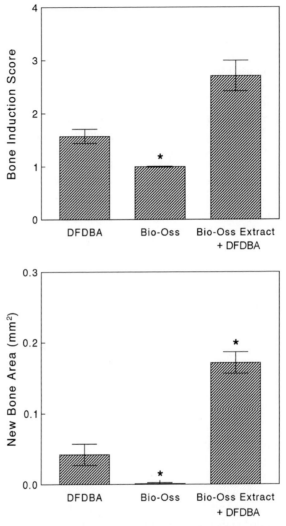

Fig. 3. Effect of Bio-Oss extracts containing BMP-2 on the ability of low-activity human DFDBA to induce bone formation in the gastrocnemius muscle of immunocompromised mice. The osteoinduction score was determined using a semiquantitative scale (*top panel*). The area of new bone was determined histomorphometrically (*bottom panel*). Values are expressed as means ± SEM for 8 implants. *, $P < 0.05$ versus DFDBA alone.

in a bone site, but those factors that inhibit osteoinduction may have usefulness orthotopically as long as the site is not overly compromised.

• Simply adding a growth factor or cell attachment ligand may be sufficient in fresh fractures in healthy rats but may not be effective in patients, especially when confounding variables are present, in particular those involving age and pharmacology.

- The rate of graft resorption may be a critical variable depending on the intended use of a material and should be considered when designing any kind of bone graft substitute.
- Each bioactive factor acts through a distinct mechanism that influences its relative function when used clinically. Understanding those mechanisms is important when selecting a material for a specific application.

Acknowledgments

The authors thank the many companies that have provided support for these studies.

References

[1] Reddi AH. Implant-stimulated interface reactions during collagenous bone matrix-induced bone formation. J Biomed Mater Res 1985;19:233–9.
[2] Urist MR. Bone: formation by autoinduction. Science 1965;150:893–9.
[3] Dragoo JL, Lieberman JR, Lee RS, et al. Tissue-engineered bone from BMP-2-transduced stem cells derived from human fat. Plast Reconstr Surg 2005;115:1665–73.
[4] Schreiber RE, Blease K, Ambrosio A, et al. Bone induction by AdBMP-2/collagen implants. J Bone Joint Surg Am 2005;87:1059–68.
[5] Fiorellini JP, Howell TH, Cochran D, et al. Randomized study evaluating recombinant human bone morphogenetic protein-2 for extraction socket augmentation. J Periodontol 2005; 76:605–13.
[6] Wozney JM. Overview of bone morphogenetic proteins. Spine 2002;27(16 Suppl. 1):S2–8.
[7] Granjeiro JM, Oliveira RC, Bustos-Valenzuela JC, et al. Bone morphogenetic proteins: from structure to clinical use. Braz J Med Biol Res 2005;38:1463–73.
[8] Behnam K, Brochmann E, Murray S. Alkali-urea extraction of demineralized bone matrix removes noggin, an inhibitor of bone morphogenetic proteins. Connect Tissue Res 2004; 45:257–60.
[9] Yanagita M. BMP antagonists: their roles in development and involvement in pathophysiology. Cytokine Growth Factor Rev 2005;16:309–17.
[10] Schwartz Z, Mellonig JT, Carnes DL Jr, et al. Ability of commercial demineralized freeze-dried bone allograft to induce new bone formation. J Periodontol 1996;67:918–26.
[11] Schwartz Z, Somers A, Mellonig JT, et al. Ability of commercial demineralized freeze-dried bone allograft to induce new bone formation is dependent on donor age but not gender. J Periodontol 1998;69:470–8.
[12] Schwartz Z, Weesner T, van Dijket S, et al. Ability of deproteinized cancellous bovine bone to induce new bone formation. J Periodontol 2000;71:1258–69.
[13] Ranly DM, McMillan J, Keller T, et al. Platelet-derived growth factor inhibits demineralized bone matrix-induced intramuscular cartilage and bone formation. A study of immunocompromised mice. J Bone Joint Surg [Am] 2005;87:2052–64.
[14] Weibrich G, Kleis WK, Buch R, et al. The Harvest Smart PRePTM system versus the Friadent-Schutze platelet-rich plasma kit. Clin Oral Implants Res 2003;14:233–9.
[15] Ranly DM, McMillan J, Keller T, et al. Platelet-derived growth factor inhibits demineralized bone matrix-induced intramuscular cartilage and bone formation. A study of immunocompromised mice. J Bone Joint Surg [Am] 2005;87:2052–64.
[16] Zhang M, Powers RM Jr, Wolfinbarger L Jr. A quantitative assessment of osteoinductivity of human demineralized bone matrix. J Periodontol 1997;68:1076–84.
[17] Venezia E, Goldstein M, Boyan BD, et al. The use of enamel matrix derivative in the treatment of periodontal defects: a literature review and meta-analysis. Crit Rev Oral Biol Med 2004;15:382–402.

[18] Suzuki S, Nagano T, Yamakoshi Y, et al. Enamel matrix derivative gel stimulates signal transduction of BMP and TGF-β. J Dent Res 2005;84:510–4.

[19] Schwartz Z, Carnes DL Jr, Pulliam R, et al. Porcine fetal enamel matrix derivative stimulates proliferation but not differentiation of pre-osteoblastic 2T9 cells, inhibits proliferation and stimulates differentiation of osteoblast-like MG63 cells, and increases proliferation and differentiation of normal human osteoblast NHOst cells. J Periodontol 2000;71:1287–96.

[20] Shimizu E, Saito R, Nakayama Y, et al. Amelogenin stimulates bone sialoprotein (BSP) expression through fibroblast growth factor 2 response element and transforming growth factor-beta1 activation Element in the promoter of the BSP gene. J Periodontol 2005;76:1482–9.

[21] Williams LT, Escobedo JA, Keating MT, et al. The stimulation of paracrine and autocrine mitogenic pathways by the platelet-derived growth factor receptor. J Cell Physiol Suppl 1987;(Suppl 5):27–30.

[22] Ranly DM, McMillan J, Keller T, et al. Platelet-derived growth factor inhibits demineralized bone matrix-induced intramuscular cartilage and bone formation. A study of immunocompromised mice. J Bone Joint Surg Am 2005;87:2052–64.

[23] Camelo M, Nevins ML, Schenk RK, et al. Periodontal regeneration in human Class II furcations using purified recombinant human platelet-derived growth factor-BB (rhPDGF-BB) with bone allograft. Int J Periodontics Restorative Dent 2003;23:213–25.

[24] Baylink DJ, Finkelman RD, Mohan S. Growth factors to stimulate bone formation. J Bone Miner Res 1993;8(Suppl 2):S565–72.

[25] Bonewald LF, Kester MB, Schwartz Z, et al. Effects of combining transforming growth factor β and 1,25-dihydroxyvitamin D_3 on differentiation of a human osteosarcoma (MG-63). J Biol Chem 1992;267:8943–9.

[26] Boyan BD, Schwartz Z, Park-Snyderet S, et al. Latent transforming growth factor-β is produced by chondrocytes and activated by extracellular matrix vesicles upon exposure to 1, 25-$(OH)_2D_3$. J Biol Chem 1994;269:28374–81.

[27] Grageda E, Lozada JL, Boyne PJ, et al. Bone formation in the maxillary sinus by using platelet-rich plasma: an experimental study in sheep. J Oral Implantol 2005;31:2–17.

[28] Marden LJ, Fan RS, Pierce GF, et al. Platelet-derived growth factor inhibits bone regeneration induced by osteogenin, a bone morphogenetic protein, in rat craniotomy defects. J Clin Invest 1993;92:2897–905.

[29] Jensen TB, Rahbek O, Overgaard S, et al. No effect of platelet-rich plasma with frozen or processed bone allograft around noncemented implants. Int Orthop 2005;29:67–72.

[30] Pryor ME, Polimeni G, Koo KT, et al. Analysis of rat calvaria defects implanted with a platelet-rich plasma preparation: histologic and histometric observations. J Clin Periodontol 2005;32:966–72.

[31] Xiao ZS, Liu SG, Hinson TK, et al. Characterization of the upstream mouse Cbfa1/Runx2 promoter. J Cell Biochem 2001;82:647–59.

[32] Boyan BD, Lohmann CH, Somers A, et al. Potential of porous poly-D, L-lactide-co-glycolide (PLG) particles as a carrier for recombinant human bone morphogenetic protein-2 during osteoinduction in vivo. J Biomed Mater Res 1999;46:51–9.

[33] Vaccaro AR, Patel T, Fischgrund J, et al. A pilot study evaluating the safety and efficacy of OP-1 Putty (rhBMP-7) as a replacement for iliac crest autograft in posterolateral lumbar arthrodesis for degenerative spondylolisthesis. Spine 2004;29:1885–92.

[34] Wildemann B, Kadow-Romacker A, Lubberstedt M, et al. Differences in the fusion and resorption activity of human osteoclasts after stimulation with different growth factors released from a polylactide carrier. Calcif Tissue Int 2005;76:50–5.

[35] Bonar LC, Glimcher MJ. Thermal denaturation of mineralized and demineralized bone collagens. J Ultrastruct Res 1970;32:545–57.

[36] Boyan BD, Weesner TC, Lohmann CH, et al. Porcine fetal enamel matrix derivative enhances bone formation induced by demineralized freeze dried bone allograft in vivo. J Periodontol 2000;71:1278–86.

ELSEVIER
SAUNDERS

THE DENTAL
CLINICS
OF NORTH AMERICA

Dent Clin N Am 50 (2006) 229–244

Reconstructive Materials and Bone Tissue Engineering in Implant Dentistry

James C. Earthman, PhD[a,b,c,*], Yong Li, PhD[b],
Lindsey R. VanSchoiack, MS[a],
Cherilyn G. Sheets, DDS[d], Jean C. Wu, DDS[d]

[a]Department of Biomedical Engineering, University of California, Irvine, CA, USA
[b]Department of Chemical Engineering and Materials Science, University of California,
Irvine, CA, USA
[c]Department of Orthopaedic Surgery, University of California, Irvine, CA, USA
[d]Newport Coast Oral-Facial Institute, Newport Beach, CA, USA

Periodontal function for natural teeth and dental implants depends strongly on the mechanical integrity of the bone in the maxilla and mandible. Ongoing healthy bone remodeling around a natural tooth or implant is critical for longevity. Chemical factors that influence bone remodeling have been explored with the goal of enhancing the growth and maintenance of good quality bone [1]. Less, but increasing, effort has been directed at understanding the mechanical signals and factors, including implant/prosthesis materials that transmit loads directly to the surrounding bone. This article reviews research on the effects of synthetic materials and resulting mechanical stimuli on bone tissue engineering in dentistry.

Effect of mechanical stresses on bone remodeling

Natural teeth and implants are subjected to loading conditions that can have a dramatic effect on the health of tissues, particularly in the case of bone. Although periodontal forces can be applied slowly or can be static under certain conditions, they are most often dynamic in situations in which mechanical stresses are repeated and relatively high loading rates are imposed. Dynamic forces can result from occlusion, such as chewing hard

* Corresponding author. Department of Chemical Engineering and Materials Science, 916 Engineering Tower, University of California, Irvine, CA 92697-2575.
E-mail address: earthman@uci.edu (J.C. Earthman).

foods and parafunctional activity, and from traumatic impact by a foreign object. These forces are generated by muscular contraction and the kinetic energy associated with the impacting bodies. In contrast, static occlusal forces normally result from prolonged muscle contraction only. The additional kinetic energy associated with dynamic forces depends on the mass and relatively high velocity of the bodies involved. For occlusion, the kinetic energy is roughly equal to the mass of the mandible multiplied by the square of its velocity relative to the maxilla. Upon impact, this velocity decelerates to zero as the kinetic energy is converted to mechanical energy and heat by energy dissipative processes. The mechanical energy gives rise to dynamic forces that add to the quasi-static forces produced by muscle contraction. As a result of normal function and parafunctional activity, these dynamic loads are repeated many times over extended periods and can give rise to fatigue damage in a tooth, dental prosthesis, or supporting bone. Dynamic forces are generally more deleterious to a structure than static loads, even when they are of lower amplitude [2,3].

Dynamic forces can provide the necessary repeated mechanical stimulus for reinforcing tissue growth that reduces the risk of fatigue failure [4]. Wolff [5] is generally given credit for first recognizing that mechanical forces are responsible for the architecture of bone. His "law of bone transformation" implied a mathematical relationship between mechanical stress and the directions of bone formation. Building on this law, Fung [6] proposed a biomechanical stress–growth relationship, which asserted that stable bone growth occurs under an intermediate range of stresses (Fig. 1) and tissue resorption results at the low (atrophy) and high (damage) extremes. In deriving this relationship, it was recognized that (1) transport of matter depends on strain of the cell membranes, (2) actin-myosin cross-bridges in the cell membranes are sensitive to strain, and (3) chemical reaction rates within the cell depend on the stress level.

Fung proposed an optimal stress level that induces a maximum growth rate. This hypothesis implies that bone loss can result from either excessively low or high stress levels (see Fig. 1). Muscle and bone have been shown to atrophy during periods of immobility and relatively low skeletal loading

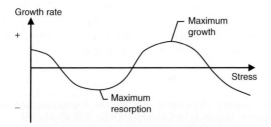

Fig. 1. Fung's stress-growth relationship. (*From* Fung YC. Biomechanics: motion, flow, stress, and growth. New York: Springer-Verlag; 1990. p. 530; with permission.)

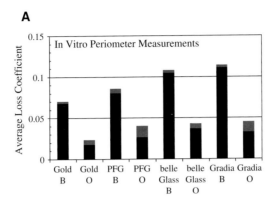

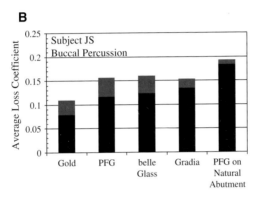

Fig. 6. Average loss coefficient for different superstructure materials and percussion directions for an in vitro implant model (*A*) and human subject (*B*). The shaded portions of the columns represent the standard deviations, and the height of the black columns indicates the average values of the loss coefficient. Columns designated with a "B" correspond to percussion in the buccal direction, and columns designated with on "O" correspond to percussion in the occlusal direction. PFG, porcelain fused to gold. (*From* Barzin A, Sheets CG, Earthman JC. Mechanical biocompatibility of dental implant materials. In: Proceedings of the 4th Pacific Rim International Conference on Advanced Materials and Processing (PRICM4). Sendai (Japan): The Japan Institute of Metals; 2001. p. 2952; with permission.)

which was positioned between the post and the submucosal part of the implant, was characterized as two linear elastic materials with two different values of Young's modulus. For the freestanding implant, their results show that the static stress distribution does not change significantly during static loading when the elastic modulus of the stress-absorbing element was increased from 150 to 110,000 MPa (ie, from a soft material to a rigid material). This result implied that the primary effect that a stress-absorbing element has on bone is not related to its elastic modulus but rather to its viscous damping properties. In the case of a tooth-connected implant, the influence of the stress-absorbing element on the loading of the natural tooth was signified by a decrease of 20% to 45% in the height of the peak stresses (ie, the stress distribution becomes more uniform when stress-absorbing elements are used) [14]. A principal conclusion is that a stress-absorbing element should not be modeled simply by a linear elastic material. Rather, a realistic model should include a damping capacity term for this element that characterizes dissipation of mechanical energy during dynamic loading.

More recently, Genna and colleagues [26] studied the behavior of a PDL-like layer using three-dimensional finite element analysis. In their paper, nonlinear hyperelastic deformation was assumed for the PDL-like layer, and they found that such an implant can be effective in terms of stress redistribution and stress absorption even in the case of a freestanding implant. They also noted that the PDL layer helps to reduce significantly the axial stress in the connecting screw caused by its tightening and the self-stresses induced by geometric misfits. It is evident from the results of van Rossen and colleagues [14] and Genna and colleagues [26] that the damping capacity of the PDL plays a crucial role in redistributing and absorbing dynamic stresses transmitted through teeth into bone. An implant material that mimics the damping capacity provided by the PDL would be of interest to enhance the longevity and reliability of the implant structures.

Few efforts have been made to identify and develop high damping materials to serve the purpose of dental implantation. Among those materials, commercially available polymers, such as polymethyl methacrylate and polyoxymethylene, have been used because they have higher damping capacities than almost all metals. Ironically, polymer elements that reduce damage to the bone and other components of the implant structure tend to fail by fatigue after relatively short periods, which results in frequent replacement. Consequently, the limited fatigue resistance of these materials has hindered their widespread use as PDL-like elements [27]. New designs are being developed that attempt to address this problem. For example, Gaggl and Schultes [28] proposed an implant structure that they claim is maintenance free and contains silicone rings. It remains to be seen whether the longevity of the polymer elements in this and other new designs is comparable to the metallic materials in use.

Commercially pure titanium has been considered one of the most chemically biocompatible materials [29]. These materials generally have much better fatigue properties than those of polymers but also have high elastic moduli and low damping capacities compared with bone. A mismatch in elastic modulus is often cited as the mechanical factor that results in poor biocompatibility because of a nonuniform stress distribution [30]. The lack of energy dissipation on the part of metallic materials can give rise to more severe problems, however, such as fatigue failure and tooth intrusion [3,15,18].

Superelastic Ti-Ni alloys have drawn considerable attention for dental applications because of their excellent corrosion resistance, superelasticity, and shape memory characteristics [31–35]. Superelasticity results from the stress-induced phase transformation that is characterized by a plateau in the stress versus strain response (Fig. 7). Orthodontic Ti-Ni wires stressed

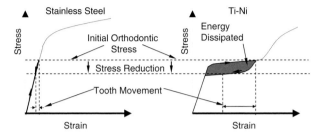

Fig. 7. Comparison of stress strain curves for stainless steel and a superelastic Ti-Ni alloy that ex-hibits a plateau resulting from stress-induced phase transformation. After an applied orthodontic stress, more tooth movement can be accommodated by a Ti-Ni wire compared with a stainless steel wire for a given decrease in applied stress. This schematic also illustrates the energy dissipation that is achieved by the Ti-Ni alloy when deforming in the superelastic plateau region.

into the plateau region can accommodate large tooth movement (strain) with relatively little reduction in stress. Ti-Ni wires offer the advantage of fewer retightening procedures compared with stainless steel wires for a given amount of tooth movement.

Iramaneerat and colleagues [34] investigated dynamic force transmission during orthodontic archwire application using dynamic finite element analysis. Their results showed that the superelastic Ti-Ni alloy wire has a damping capacity that is more than twice that of a stainless steel wire counterpart. This additional damping on the part of Ti-Ni caused by irreversible phase transformation is also shown schematically in Fig. 7. More quantitatively, De Santis and colleagues [36] reported a damping coefficient of approximately 0.004 for a Ti-Ni alloy at a high frequency of approximately 300 Hz. When used in orthodontic archwire applications, it has been shown that superelastic Ti-Ni wire has the ability to buffer a significant amount of the dynamic occlusal force transmitted to the PDL [37]. This finding is consistent with the results in Fig. 3, which show the sizable reduction in transmitted occlusal loads that can be accomplished with a modest increase in the damping capacity of the structure.

The cytotoxicity of Ni has been a concern for Ti-Ni alloys used for implants [27], and extensive efforts in surface modification are still being made to address the issue [38]. Accordingly, the use of Ti-Ni in its current compositions is generally not recommended for dental implants. Its use in abutments and superstructures above the tissue level, as in the case of orthodontic wires, should be acceptable, however. The ultimate goal is to achieve a combination of longevity, energy dissipation, and aesthetics that has so far eluded many researchers and clinicians.

Immediate loading of implants and bone remodeling

Immediate loading refers to the fixation of a prosthesis to an implant in or out of direct occlusal function within 48 hours of surgical placement.

There are several categories of immediately loaded implants. First, an implant can be placed into healed bone where the initial stability depends predominately on the surgical technique, bone density, bone height, and implant geometry. Second, an implant can be placed immediately into a fresh extraction site, which adds further complications to establishing initial stability. The complicating factors include the size of the extracted tooth versus the size of the implant replacement, density of the surrounding bone, potential need for grafting, presence of micro- or macrofractures of the bone complex from the extraction process itself, and the potential presence of infection associated with the extracted tooth that could jeopardize the osseointegration process. For successful osseointegration, both situations depend highly on being protected from excess forces during the initial healing process. It is believed that the most damaging forces on the immediately placed implant are from excessive postsurgical loading from parafunctional habit patterns and unmonitored mastication [39].

Convention has established that traditional methods of determining implant stability, such as the tapping of an implant fixture with the end of a mouth mirror and radiographs, are sufficient indicators of implant health. Certainly high success rates for implants in both arches are documented in the literature. A growing number of scientists and clinicians are starting to call for systems that provide a more definitive measurement of osseointegration, however [40–50].

The ability to quantify levels of osseointegration is important because of two current trends in implant dentistry. First, the traditional Brånemark two-stage placement protocol has been modified toward immediate or early loading of implants. An increase in the number of osseointegration failures is anticipated as more high-risk immediate load surgeries are performed. Several authors are reporting early indications of this disturbing possibility [51–53]. Second, there is an increasing trend to train nonspecialists to place and restore implants [54]. Although there are many good reasons to expand the number of clinicians who provide implant services, it does place less experienced clinicians in the roles that formerly have been held by trained specialists.

The intersection of these two trends has the potential of creating an environment of increasing implant failures. Quantitative methods of assessing osseointegration and fixture structural integrity must be introduced into accepted protocols. Quantitative monitoring of implants allows therapeutic measures to be instituted when implants become vulnerable to disintegration [39]. Currently, therapeutic measures are not instituted until bone loss can be identified by radiographs or clinical mobility, which is often too late in the failure process to establish implant health.

Ideally, a clinician should be able to obtain sensitive biomechanical information critical to implant health and longevity in a nondestructive, cost-effective, and noninvasive manner. A system also should be able to provide information throughout all stages of implant life—information that would allow early effective therapeutic intervention when indicated.

Biomechanical approaches for assessing implant and bone stability

The most commonly used method for assessing implant stability is the use of manual percussion and the subsequent evaluation of the auditory sound. Numerous authors have described the lack of discernment that this method provides [55]. Although gross levels of osseointegration can be assessed in this way, there is no ability to determine levels of osseointegration or bone quality. Numerous experimental models have been noted in the literature, few of which have become commercially viable and have been relegated to limited research use at best. Two exceptions are a unit that measures percussion time (Periotest [MedizinTechnik Gulden, Lautertal, Germany]) and a unit that measures resonance frequency (Osstell Mentor [Integration Diagnostics AB, Göteborg, Sweden]).

The Periotest unit was designed to measure periodontal stability of natural teeth. The instrument measures percussion time on an arbitrary scale and is expressed in Periotest values. The Periotest has provided some information for evaluation of the osseointegration process in the literature but has not received widespread acceptance for several reasons [56]. The most damaging criticism is that the Periotest gives inconsistent results. The inconsistency has been related to several factors: the probe must be held steady in a horizontal position so that the tip is 2 mm from the surface of the implant, the unit is not shielded from external electromagnetic noise, and the resolution of the Periotest values scale is limited in the range corresponding to implants [43,44,55,57].

The Osstell Mentor uses the measurement of resonance frequency as an indicator of implant stability. The new version of this technology recently was released in Europe. The Osstell system provides a more quantitative and reliable measurement of implant stability compared with the Periotest. The Osstell also has limitations, however: a specialized measuring device ("smart peg") must be attached directly to the implant at the fixture level, each implant design requires a different smart peg geometry for testing, it is inconvenient to disassemble the implant for each testing session, the act of disassembly can compromise the mucosal barrier and result in the loss of connective tissue and bone during the early stages of implant healing, and the measurements are subject to some variability because of differences in bone quality [58,59]. Accordingly, this system has not realized widespread acceptance in the United States.

A more recently developed system that measures the structural stability and integrity for dental implants and natural teeth is the Periometer (Perimetrics, LLC, Newport Beach, California). This device provides two pieces of diagnostic information: the loss coefficient of the structure (described previously) and an energy return time profile that indicates localized defects, such as cracks and loose fixtures. The analysis of these two results gives a wealth of information regarding the attachment of an implant to the bone and the structural stability of the entire implant complex being tested.

The features of this device are a handheld probe, a disposable stabilization tip, a horizontal level scale, a computer interface, data analysis software, statistical validity indicators, automatic abnormal analysis and alerts, and a medical grade power supply and shielding. The Periometer is able to gather diagnostic data at every stage of implant life using clinically relevant mechanical energy. It does not induce an artificial strain rate and provides two related categories of diagnostic information: the loss coefficient and energy return profile. The Periometer is currently being used for research at the University of California, Irvine, California; the Newport Coast Oral-Facial Institute in Newport Beach, California; and the Veterans Administration Medical Center, San Diego, California.

Tissue engineering research for tooth replacement

The ultimate solution for dental tooth loss is the actual fabrication of complex tooth structures by some method of tissue engineering to produce a biologic tooth substitute. Globally, many research teams are working to understand odontogenesis. The three main areas of focus are the tissue cells to be generated, the extracellular matrix, and the scaffolding on which the tissues grow. Artificial scaffolds lack critical cell signaling capabilities and can interfere with new tissue growth. Natural biodegradable materials, such as collagen, alginate, and silk, can be used to create scaffolds that are compatible with the desired cell and tissue functions and are eventually biodegradable. Understanding the molecular mechanisms that control tooth development can help identify the developmental processes that control tooth shape, tooth number, and cuspal development.

Structurally correct teeth have been grown by several approaches, including building teeth from existing dental cells or growing them from progenitor tissues [60–63]. Remaining challenges include growing roots and identifying ideal raw materials for bioengineered human teeth. Progress has been achieved to the point that many researchers believe that test-tube teeth may become the first engineered organs.

Young and colleagues [60] dissociated porcine and rat tooth buds into single-cell suspensions and seeded them onto biodegradable polymer scaffolds [63]. As demonstrated in Fig. 8, rat hosts produced recognizable tooth structures that contained dentin, odontoblasts, a well-defined pulp chamber, putative Hertwig's root sheath epithelia, putative cementoblasts, and a morphologically correct enamel organ. This was the first successful generation of tooth crowns from dissociated tooth tissues that contained dentin and enamel and suggested the presence of epithelial and mesenchymal dental stem cells in porcine and rat tooth bud tissues.

Despite these remarkable achievements, the bioengineered teeth were still small and did not conform to the scaffolds. It should be noted that the scaffolds were implanted into the omentum as opposed to the mandible or maxilla. Inadequate mechanical stimulus could have been one of the factors that

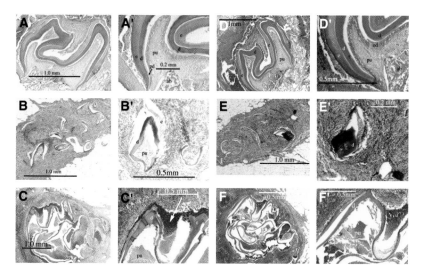

Fig. 8. Histologic analysis of scaffolds that contain rat tooth bud cells after 12 weeks of implantation in the omentum. Positive control intact tooth bud implants exhibited dentin, enamel, and pulp tissues (*A, A'*). Dental cell seeded in biodegradable polyglycolic acid (*B, B'*) and polylactic co-glycolic acid (*C, C'*) scaffold tooth tissues also generated dentin, enamel, and pulp tissues. Infiltrating lymphocytes were occasionally observed in dental implants (*C, C'*) (*arrow*). Goldner's stain of positive control intact tooth bud implants revealed blue-stained dentin, red-stained immature enamel, and gray-stained mature enamel (*D, D'*). Polyglycolic acid– and polylactic co-glycolic acid–bioengineered teeth exhibited blue-stained dentin, whereas polyglycolic acid generally produced mature, gray-stained enamel at 12 weeks, and polylactic co-glycolic acid generated red- and gray-stained mature enamel (*E, E', F, F'*). d, dentin; e, enamel; em, enamel matrix; pe, pre-enamel; pu, pulp. (*From* Duailibi MT, Duailibi SE, Young CS, et al. Bioengineered teeth from cultured rat tooth bud cells. J Dent Res 2004;83(7):592; with permission.)

led to the observed deficiency in tooth formation. The authors cited the need to better understand cell–scaffold interactions and the underlying mechanisms that direct the growth of the tooth tissues [60,63]. As evidenced by the works reviewed in this article, dynamic loading plays an important role in these mechanisms. A greater understanding of the role that mechanical loading plays in governing tissue formation and remodeling must continue to be achieved if tissue engineering in general is to reach its full potential.

References

[1] Ueda M, Tohnai I, Nakai H. Tissue engineering research in oral implant surgery. Artif Organs 2001;25(3):164–71.

[2] Burr DB. Bone exercise and stress fractures. Exerc Sport Sci Rev 1997;25:171–94.

[3] Duyck J, Rønold HJ, Oosterwyck HV, et al. The influence of static and dynamic loading on marginal bone reactions around osseointegrated implants: an animal experimental study. Clin Oral Implants Res 2001;12:207–18.

[4] Martin RB, Burr BD, Sharkey NA. Skeletal tissue mechanics. New York: Springer-Verlag; 1998.

[5] Wolff J. Das gesetz der transformation der knochen [The law of the transformation of bone]. Berlin (Germany): Hirschwald; 1892 [in German].

[6] Fung YC. Biomechanics: motion, flow, stress, and growth. New York: Springer-Verlag; 1990.

[7] Vaughan J. The physiology of bone. New York: Oxford University Press; 1981.

[8] Takakuda K. A hypothetical regulation mechanism of adaptive bone remodeling. JSME International Journal 1993;36:417–24.

[9] Owan I, Burr DB, Turner CH, et al. Mechanotransduction in bone: osteoblasts are more responsive to fluid forces than mechanical strain. Am J Phys 1997;273:C810–5.

[10] Rubin J, McLeod KJ, Titus L, et al. Formation of osteoclast-like cells is suppressed by low frequency, low intensity electric fields. J Orthop Res 1996;14:7–15.

[11] McLeod KJ, Rubin CT, Otter MW, et al. Skeletal cell stresses and bone adaptation. Am J Med Sci 1998;316:176–83.

[12] Ogasawara A, Arakawa T, Kaneda T, et al. Fluid shear stress-induced cyclooxygenase-2 expression is mediated by C/EBP b, cAMP-response element-binding protein, and AP-1 in osteoblastic MC3T3–E1 cells. J Biol Chem 2001;276:7048–54.

[13] Chapman RJ, Kirsch A. Variations in occlusal forces with a resilient internal implant shock absorber. Int J Oral Maxillofac Implants 1990;5:369–74.

[14] Van Rossen IP, Braak LH, De Putter C, et al. Stress-absorbing elements in dental-implants. J Prosthet Dent 1990;64:198–205.

[15] Sheets CG, Earthman JC. Natural tooth intrusion and reversal in implant assisted prosthesis: evidence of and a hypothesis for the occurrence. J Prosthet Dent 1993;70:513–20.

[16] El Charkawi HG, Zekry KA, El Wakad MT. Stress analysis of different osseointegrated implants supporting a distal extension prosthesis. J Prosthet Dent 1994;72:614–22.

[17] Katona TR, Paydar NH, Akay HU, et al. Stress analysis of bone modeling response to rat molar orthodontics. J Biomech 1995;28:27–38.

[18] Sheets CG, Earthman JC. Tooth intrusion in implant-assisted prostheses. J Prosthet Dent 1997;77:39–45.

[19] Mensor MC, Ahlstrom RH, Scheerer EW. Compliant keeper system replication of the periodontal ligament protective damping function for implants. Part I. J Prosthet Dent 1998;80:565–9.

[20] Taylor D, Lee CT. A crack growth model for the simulation of fatigue in bone. Int J Fatigue 2003;25:387–95.

[21] Ödman J, Lekholm U, Jemt T, et al. Osseointegrated implants as orthodontic anchorage in the treatment of partially edentulous adult patients. Eur J Orthod 1994;16:187–201.

[22] El-Homsi F, Lockowandt P, Linden L. Simulating periodontal effects in dental osseointegrated implants: effect of an intramobile damping element on the fatigue strength of dental implants. An in vitro test method. Quintessence Int 2004;35:449–55.

[23] Barzin A, Sheets CG, Earthman JC. Mechanical biocompatibility of dental implant materials. In: Proceedings of the 4th Pacific Rim International Conference on Advanced Materials and Processing (PRICM4). Sendai (Japan): The Japan Institute of Metals; 2001. p. 2949–52.

[24] Chapman RJ, Kirsch A. Variations in occlusal forces with a resilient internal implant shock absorber. Int J Oral Maxillofac Implants 1990;5:369–74.

[25] Haas R, Bernhart T, Dortbudak O, et al. Experimental study of the damping behaviour of IMZ implants. J Oral Rehabil 1999;26:19–24.

[26] Genna F, Paranelli C, Salgarello S, et al. 3–D numerical analysis of the stress state caused by short-term loading of a fixed dental implant containing a "PDL-like" nonlinear elastic internal layer. Computer Modeling in Engineering and Sciences 2003;4:405–20.

[27] Ow RKK, Ho KH. Retrieval of the resilient element in an osseointegrated implant system. J Prosthet Dent 1992;68:93–5.

[28] Gaggl A, Schultes G. Biomechanical properties in titanium implants with integrated maintenance free shock absorbing elements. Biomaterials 2001;22:3061–6.

[29] Niimoni M. Recent metallic materials for biomedical applications. Metallurgical and Materials Transactions 2002;33A:477–86.

[30] Papavasiliou G, Kamposiora P, Bayne SC, et al. Three-dimensional finite element analysis of stress-distribution around single tooth implants as a function of bony support, prosthesis type, and loading during function. J Prosthet Dent 1996;76:633–40.

[31] Andreasen G, Hilleman T. An evaluation of 55 cobalt substituted Nitinol wire for use in orthodontics. J Am Dent Assoc 1971;82:1373–5.

[32] Gil FJ, Solano E, Peña J, et al. Microstructural, mechanical and citotoxicity evaluation of different NiTi and NiTiCu shape memory alloys. J Mater Sci Mater Med 2004;15:1181–5.

[33] Shabalovaskaya SA. Physicochemical and biological aspects of Nitinol as a biomaterial. Int Materials Rev 2001;46:233–50.

[34] Iramaneerat K, Hisano M, Soma K. Dynamic analysis for clarifying occlusal force transmission during orthodontic archwire application: difference between ISW and stainless steel. J Med Dent Sci 2004;51:59–65.

[35] Auricchio F, Petrini L, Pietrabissa R, et al. Numerical modeling of shape-memory alloys in orthodontics. CMES Computer Modeling in Engineering & Science 2003;4:365–80.

[36] De Santis S, Trochu SF, Ostiguy G. Stress-strain hysteresis and damping in MnCu and NiTi alloys. Metallurgical and Materials Transactions 2001;32A:2489–98.

[37] Lammering R, Schmidt I. Experimental investigations on the damping capacity of NiTi components. Smart Mater Struct 2001;10:853–9.

[38] Shabalovaskaya SA. Surface, corrosion and biocompatibility aspects of Nitinol as an implant material. Biomed Mater Eng 2002;12:69–109.

[39] Glauser R, Sennerby L, Meredith N, et al. Resonance frequency analysis of implants subjected to immediate or early functional occlusal loading. Clin Oral Implants Res 2004; 15(4):428–34.

[40] Oka H, Yamamoto T, Saratani K, et al. Automatic diagnosis system of tooth mobility for clinical use. Med Prog Technol 1990;16:117–24.

[41] Elias JJ, Brunski JB, Scarton HA. A dynamic modal testing technique for noninvasive assessment of bone-dental implant interfaces. Int J Oral Maxillofac Implants 1996;11(6):728–34.

[42] Olsson M, Urde G, Andersen JB, et al. Early loading of maxillary fixed cross-arch dental prostheses supported by six or eight oxidized titanium implants: results after 1 year of loading. Case series. Clin Implant Dent Relat Res 2003;5(Suppl 1):81–7.

[43] Ramp LC, Jeffcoat RL. Dynamic behavior of implants as a measure of osseointegration. Int J Oral Maxillofac Implants 2001;16(5):637–45.

[44] Geurs NC, Jeffcoat RL, McGlumphy EA, et al. Influence of implant geometry and surface characteristics on progressive osseointegration. Int J Oral Maxillofac Implants 2002;17(6): 811–5.

[45] Jeffcoat RL, Hathcoat BJ, Johnson GC. 1275 implantable biomechanical impedance sensing of osseointegration: validation in vitro. Presented at the Annual Conference of the International Association for Dental Research. San Diego (California), March 4–8, 2002.

[46] Meredith N, Alleyne D, Cawley P. Quantitative determination of the stability of the implant-tissue interface using resonance frequency analysis. Clin Oral Implants Res 1996; 7(3):261–7.

[47] Rasmusson L, Meredith N, Kahnberg KE, et al. Stability assessments and histology of titanium implants placed simultaneously with autogenous onlay bone in the rabbit tibia. Int J Oral Maxillofac Surg 1998;27:229–35.

[48] Cawley P, Pavlakovic B, Alleyne DN, et al. The design of a vibration transducer to monitor the integrity of dental implants. Proc Inst Mech Eng [H] 1998;212(4):265–72.

[49] Heo SJ, Sennerby L, Odersjo M, et al. Stability measurements of craniofacial implants by means of resonance frequency analysis: a clinical pilot study. J Laryngol Otol 1998;112(6): 537–42.

[50] O'Sullivan D, Sennerby L, Meredith N. Measurements comparing the initial stability of five designs of dental implants: a human cadaver study. Clin Implant Dent Relat Res 2000;2(2): 85–92.

[51] Glauser R, Rée A, Lundgren A, et al. Immediate occlusal loading of Brånemark implants applied in various jawbone regions: a prospective, 1-year study. Clin Implant Res 2001; 3(4):204–13.

[52] Wolfinger GJ, Balshi TJ, Rangert B. Immediate functional loading of Brånemark system implants in edentulous mandibles: clinical report of the results of developmental and simplified protocols. Int J Oral Maxillofac Implants 2003;18(2):250–7.

[53] Uribe R, Peñarrocha M, Balaguer J, et al. Immediate loading in oral implant: present situation. Med Oral Patol Oral Cir Bucal 2005;10(Suppl 2):E143–53.

[54] Schlossberg M. Incorporating implants. AGD Impact 2005;32(7):14–6.

[55] Meredith N. A review of nondestructive test methods and their application to measure the stability and osseointegration of bone anchored endosseous implants. Crit Rev Biomed Eng 1998;26(4):275–91.

[56] Winkler S, Morris HF, Spray JR. Stability of implants and natural teeth as determined by the Periotest over 60 months of function. J Oral Implantology 2001;27(4):198–203.

[57] Meredith N, Friberg B, Sennerby L, et al. Relationship between contact time measurements and PTV values when using the Periotest to measure implant stability. Int J Prosthodont 1998;11(3):269–75.

[58] Rocci A, Martigononi M, Burgos PM, et al. Histology of retrieved immediately and early loaded oxidized implants: light microscopic observations after 5 to 9 months of loading in the posterior mandible. Clin Implant Dent Relat Res 2003;5(Suppl 1):88–98.

[59] Abrahamsson I, Berglundh T, Lindhe J. The mucosal barrier following abutment dis/reconnection: an experimental study in dogs. J Clin Periodontol 1997;24:568–72.

[60] Young CS, Terada S, Vacanti JP, et al. Tissue engineering of complex tooth structures on biodegradable polymer scaffolds. J Dent Res 2002;81(10):695–700.

[61] Chai Y, Slavkin HC. Prospects for tooth generation in the 21st century: a perspective. Microsc Res Tech 2003;60(5):469–79.

[62] Ohazama A, Modino SAC, Miletich I, et al. Stem cell based tissue engineering of murine teeth. J Dent Res 2004;83(7):518–22.

[63] Duailibi MT, Duailibi SE, Young CS, et al. Bioengineered teeth from cultured rat tooth bud cells. J Dent Res 2004;83(7):523–8.

THE DENTAL
CLINICS
OF NORTH AMERICA

Dent Clin N Am 50 (2006) 245–263

Gene Therapeutics for Periodontal Regenerative Medicine

Christoph A. Ramseier, DMD[a,b],
Zachary R. Abramson, BS[a], Qiming Jin, DDS, PhD[a],
William V. Giannobile, DDS, DMedSc[a,b,c,*]

[a]Center for Craniofacial Regeneration and Department of Periodontics and Oral Medicine,
University of Michigan, Ann Arbor, MI, USA
[b]Michigan Center for Oral Health Research, University of Michigan Clinical Center,
Ann Arbor, MI, USA
[c]Department of Biomedical Engineering, College of Engineering, University of Michigan,
Ann Arbor, MI, USA

Current knowledge about the pathogenesis of periodontal disease—obtained mainly from the results of animal experiments, analysis of periodontal histopathology, epidemiologic studies, and clinical trials—describes a complex and multifactorial etiology [1]. Generally, the extent and severity of periodontitis increases with age and relates to the control of pathogens associated with dental plaque biofilms [2]. Periodontal disease is found with high prevalence and variability, with few individuals experiencing advanced destruction [3]. Periodontal disease is characterized by an inflammatory reaction of periodontal tissues that leads to destruction of tooth-associated structures, including alveolar bone, tooth root cementum, and periodontal ligament (PDL) [4]. Current views consider a course of the disease that is chronic with brief episodes of localized exacerbation and remission [5,6]. Consequently, if the disease is left untreated, tooth loss can occur. Despite the remarkably high standards of professional periodontal care currently available, incomplete adult dentitions or edentulism are still evident in the United States and worldwide populations.

This work was supported by National Institutes of Health/National Institute of Dental and Craniofacial Research grants RO1-DE13397, R21-DE 016619, and RO1-DE 015384 (to W.V. Giannobile).

* Corresponding author. Michigan Center for Oral Health Research, University of Michigan Clinical Center, 24 Frank Lloyd Wright Drive, Lobby M, Box 422, Ann Arbor, MI 48106.

E-mail address: wgiannob@umich.edu (W.V. Giannobile).

A challenge faced by periodontal therapy is the predictable regeneration of periodontal tissues lost as a consequence of disease, including alveolar bone, PDL, and cementum. Thus far, the ability to regenerate completely the damaged periodontal supporting structures has not been achieved in humans. The application of various regenerative biomaterials, such as bone autografts, allografts, cell occlusive barrier membranes used in guided tissue regeneration procedures, applications of growth factors (eg, enamel matrix proteins), or their combinations, have been pursued with varying degrees of success to regenerate lost tooth support, however [7]. Examples of currently available regenerative biomaterials are shown in Table 1 [8–37]. In summary, these therapeutic measures are shown to be limited in the predictability of healing and regenerative response in modern clinical practice, because the oral environment presents several complicating factors that border regeneration: (1) Periodontal wounds are contaminated with tooth-associated biofilms of anaerobic bacteria. (2) Transmucosal hard-soft tissue

Table 1
Various biomaterials available for clinical periodontal regenerative therapy

Regenerative biomaterials	Components	References
Bone allografts	Demineralized freeze dried bone allograft	Gurinsky et al, 2004 [8] Kimble et al, 2004 [9] Trejo et al, 2000 [10]
Bone xenografts	Bovine mineral matrix	Hartman et al, 2004 [11] Camelo et al, 2001 [12] Mellonig, 2000 [13] Nevins et al, 2000 [14] Richardson et al, 1999 [15]
Bone alloplast grafts	Beta tricalcium phosphate	Palti and Hoch, 2002 [16] Scher et al, 1999 [17] Nery et al, 1992 [18]
	Bioactive glass	Sculean et al, 2005 [19] Reynolds et al, 2003 [20] Trombelli et al, 2002 [21] Fetner et al, 1994 [22]
Nonresorbable cell occlusive barrier membranes	Polytetrafluorethylene	Trombelli et al, 2005 [23] Moses et al, 2005 [24] Murphy and Gunsolley, 2003 [25] Needleman et al, 2002 [26]
Resorbable cell occlusive barrier membranes	Polyglycolide/polylactide (synthetic)	Minenna et al, 2005 [27] Stavropoulos et al, 2004 [28] Parashis et al, 2003 [29]
	Collagen membrane (xenogen)	Sculean et al, 2005 [30] Owczarek et al, 2003 [31] Camelo et al, 1998 [32]
Enamel proteins	Enamel matrix derivative	Rasperini et al, 2005 [33] Rosing et al, 2005 [34] Sanz et al, 2004 [35] Francetti et al, 2004 [36] Tonetti et al, 2002 [37]

environment allows entry of pathogens into wounds. (3) Multiple junctional complexes and stromal-cellular interactions create difficulty in rebuilding tissue interfaces (eg, tooth-PDL-bone and epithelial-connective tissue-bone). (4) The effects of occlusal forces deliver intermittent loads in axial and transverse dimensions [38,39].

The role of growth factors used in periodontal regenerative medicine

After periodontal therapy (eg, deep scaling or periodontal flap surgery), a blood coagulum forms at the wound site and releases tissue growth factors locally, such as platelet-derived growth factor (PDGF) and transforming growth factor-β from degranulating platelets [40,41]. These mitogenic polypeptides attract mesenchymal cells and fibroblasts to migrate into the periodontal wound and stimulate their proliferation [42]. The continuing process of periodontal tissue repair is followed by the formation of granulation tissue as a source for future periodontal connective tissue cells, such as osteoblasts, PDL fibroblasts, and cementoblasts [43]. For alveolar bone regeneration, mesenchymal cells are induced into osteoprogenitor cells by locally expressed bone morphogenetic proteins (BMPs) [44,45].

Wound-healing approaches that use growth factors to target restoration of tooth-supporting bone, PDL, and cementum can advance greatly the field of periodontal regenerative medicine. A major focus of periodontal research has evaluated the impact of growth factor applications on periodontal tissue regeneration [39,46–48]. Articles describe various delivery systems and applications of growth factors, which are highlighted in Table 2. Advances in molecular cloning have made available unlimited quantities of recombinant growth factors for applications in tissue engineering. Recombinant growth factors known to promote skin and bone wound healing, such as PDGFs [49–53], insulin-like growth factors [46,50,54,55], fibroblast growth factors [56–60], and BMPs [61–65], have been used in preclinical and clinical

Table 2
Effects of growth factors used for periodontal tissue engineering

Growth factor	Effects
Platelet-derived growth factor	Migration, proliferation, and noncollagenous matrix synthesis of mesenchymal cells
Insulin-like growth factor-1	Cell migration, proliferation, differentiation, and matrix synthesis
Fibroblast growth factor-2	Proliferation and attachment of endothelial cells and PDL cells
Transforming growth factor-beta	Proliferation of cementoblasts and PDL fibroblasts
Bone morphogenetic protein	Differentiation of osteoblasts, differentiation of PDL cells into osteoblasts
Enamel matrix derivative	Proliferation, protein synthesis, and mineral nodule formation in PDL cells, osteoblasts, and cementoblasts

trials for the treatment of large periodontal or intrabony defects and around dental implants [66,67].

Biologic effects of growth factors: platelet-derived growth factors

PDGF is a member of a multifunctional polypeptide family that binds to two cell membrane tyrosine kinase receptors (PDGF-Rα and PDGF-Rβ) and subsequently exerts its biologic effects on cell proliferation, migration, extracellular matrix synthesis, and anti-apoptosis [68–71]. PDGF-α and -β receptors are expressed in regenerating periodontal soft and hard tissues [72]. PDGF also initiates tooth-supporting PDL cell chemotaxis [73], mito-genesis [74], matrix synthesis [75], and attachment to tooth dentinal surfaces [76]. More importantly, in vivo application of PDGF alone or in combination with insulin-like growth factor-1 results in partial repair of periodontal tissues [49,50,55,77,78]. PDGF has been shown to have a significant regenerative im-pact on PDL cells and osteoblasts [42,52,74,79].

Biologic effects of growth factors: bone morphogenetic proteins

BMPs are multifunctional polypeptides that belong to the transforming growth factor-β superfamily of proteins [80]. The human genome encodes at least 20 BMPs [81]. BMPs bind to type I and II receptors that function as serine-threonine kinases. The type I receptor protein kinase phosphory-lates intracellular signaling substrates called Smads (Sma gene in *C elegans* and Mad gene in *Drosophila*). The phosphorylated BMP-signaling Smads enter the nucleus and initiate the production of bone matrix proteins leading to bone morphogenesis. The most remarkable feature of BMPs is the ability to induce ectopic bone formation [82]. BMPs not only are powerful regula-tors of cartilage and bone formation during embryonic development and re-generation in postnatal life but also participate in the development and repair of other organs, such as the brain, kidney, and nerves [83]. Studies have demonstrated the expression of BMPs during tooth development and periodontal repair, including alveolar bone [84,85]. Investigations in animal models have shown the potential repair of alveolar bony defects using re-combinant human BMP-12 (rhBMP-12) [63] or rhBMP-2 [86,87]. In a recent clinical trial by Fiorellini and colleagues [88], rhBMP-2 delivered by a bioab-sorbable collagen sponge revealed significant bone formation in a human buccal wall defect model after tooth extraction when compared with colla-gen sponge alone. BMP-7, also known as osteogenic protein-1, stimulates bone regeneration around teeth and endosseous dental implants and in max-illary sinus floor augmentation procedures [56,89,90].

*Clinical applications of growth factors for use in
periodontal regeneration*

In general, the impact of a topical delivery of growth factors to periodon-tal wounds has shown to be promising yet insufficient for the promotion of predictable periodontal tissue engineering [48,51]. Growth factor proteins, once delivered to the target site, tend to suffer from instability and quick dilution, presumably because of proteolytic breakdown, receptor-mediated endocytosis, and solubility of the delivery vehicle [39]. Because their half-lives are significantly reduced, the period of exposure may not be sufficient to act on osteoblasts, cementoblasts, or PDL cells. Different methods of growth factor delivery must be considered [91].

Investigations for periodontal bioengineering have examined various methods of combining delivery vehicles (eg, scaffolds) with growth factors to target the defect site to optimize bioavailability [92]. The scaffolds are designed to optimize the dosage of the growth factor and control its release pattern, which may be pulsatile, constant, or time programmed [93]. The kinetics of the release and the duration of the exposure of the growth factor also may be controlled [94].

A new polymeric system was reported in an animal study by Richardson and colleagues [95] that enabled the tissue-specific delivery of two or more growth factors, with a controlled dose and rate of delivery. The dual delivery of vascular endothelial growth factor (VEGF) together with PDGF from a single, structural polymer scaffold results in the rapid formation of a mature vascular network.

Gene therapy methods investigated for periodontal tissue regeneration

The single administration of purified tissue growth factors has not been shown to be clinically effective in supporting the horizontal regeneration of periodontal tissue breakdown. This may be caused by insufficient capabilities to maintain therapeutic protein levels at the wound site and the three-dimensional architecture of the defects. Gene transfer methods may circumvent many of the limitations with protein delivery to soft tissue wounds [96,97]. The application of growth factors [45,98–100] or soluble forms of cytokine receptors [101] by gene transfer provides a greater sustainability than that of single protein application. Gene therapy may achieve greater bioavailability of growth factors within periodontal wounds, which may provide greater regenerative potential (Fig. 1).

Gene delivery methods

In general, gene therapy involves the transfer of genetic information to target cells, which enables them to synthesize a protein of interest to treat disease [102–104]. The technology can be used to treat disorders that result from single point mutations [105] or to increase protein production [106]. The preferred strategy for gene transfer depends on the required duration of protein release and the morphology of the target site. Gene transfer is accomplished through the use of viral and nonviral vectors. Examples of viral vectors are retroviruses, adenoviruses (Ad) and adeno-associated viruses

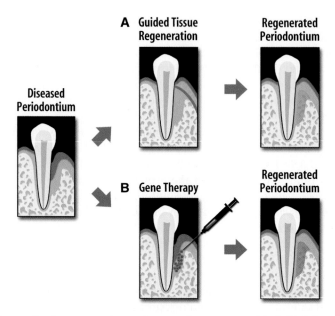

Fig. 1. Approaches for regenerating tooth-supporting structures. (*A*) Guided tissue regeneration uses a cell occlusive barrier membrane to restore periodontal tissues. (*B*) Alternatively,
an example of gene therapy uses vector-encoding growth factors aimed at stimulating the regeneration of host cells derived from the periodontium.

(AAV), and nonviral vectors include plasmids and DNA polymer complexes
(Table 3) [107].

Retroviruses introduce RNA together with two enzymes, called reverse
transcriptase and integrase, into the target cell. Initially, the reverse transcriptase enables the production of a DNA copy from the retrovirus
RNA molecule. Subsequently, the integrase adds the DNA copy into
the target cell DNA. When the genetically altered host cell divides later,
its descendants contain the modified DNA. Because the integrase enzyme
may insert the DNA copy into an arbitrary position of the target cell
DNA, gene disruption and uncontrolled cell division (ie, cancer) may
occur [107].

Ad contains DNA, which is introduced into the target cell and subsequently transferred into its nucleus. In contrast to the fate of the retrovirus DNA copy, the Ad-DNA is not incorporated into the host cell's
genetic material. Consequently, when the Ad-infected target cell divides
later, its descendants are not genetically altered, nor do they contain
the Ad-DNA genetic material [108]. AAV derive from the parvovirus
family and are small viruses with a single-stranded DNA genome that
causes no known human diseases [107–109]. The AAV infects dividing
and nondividing cells by integrating its genetic material on chromosomes
of the target cell. Types of recombinant AAV have been developed either

Table 3
Viral and nonviral gene therapy vectors used in tissue engineering

Vector	Type	Advantages/disadvantages
Retrovirus	Viral	Advantages: Nonimmunogenic Disadvantages: Infects only dividing cells Insertional mutagenesis
Adenovirus	Viral	Advantages: Infects dividing and nondividing cells Does not integrate into target cell genome Disadvantages: Potentially immunogenic
Adeno-associated virus	Viral	Advantages: Infects dividing and nondividing cells Low immunogenicity Nonpathogenic in human Disadvantages: Difficult to produce at high titers Small transgenes
Plasmid	Nonviral	Advantages: Nonimmunogenic Nonpathogenic Disadvantages: Low transduction efficiency
DNA polymer complexes	Nonviral	Advantages: Infects dividing and nondividing cells Cell-specific targeting Disadvantages: Low transduction efficiency

to remain extrachromosomal or integrate into nonspecific chromosomal sites. Research has demonstrated that the AAV can be used to correct genetic defects in animals [107,110]. One disadvantage of the AAV is that it is small and possesses the capacity to carry no more than usually two genes [109].

Because nonviral alternatives do not have the drawbacks of undesired host immune reactions or potential tumorigenesis, they likely will be given more consideration in the future. Plasmids and DNA polymer complexes carry the genetic information in the form of DNA to express a foreign protein. Design features of nonviral delivery of DNA match various requirements, such as chromosomal integration or the ability to alter gene expression [107].

Gene therapy for periodontal tissue engineering

Various gene delivery methods are available to administer growth factors to periodontal defects and offer great flexibility for tissue engineering (Fig. 2). The delivery method can be tailored to the specific characteristics

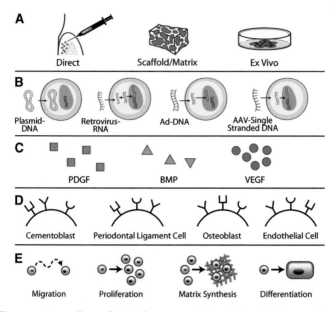

Fig. 2. The current paradigm of gene therapy used in periodontal tissue engineering. Approaches consider (*A*) methods of delivery, (*B*) gene therapy vector, (*C*) tissue growth factor, (*D*) cellular target receptors, and (*E*) local effect. The choice of delivery method, DNA vector, and growth factor should maximize expected effect, minimize patient risk, and reflect the characteristics of the wound site.

of the wound site. For example, a horizontal one- or two-walled defect may require the use of a supportive carrier, such as a scaffold. Other defect sites may be conducive to the use of an Ad vector embedded in a collagen matrix.

More important from a clinical point of view is the risk associated with the use of gene therapy in periodontal tissue engineering [111]. As with maximizing growth factor sustainability and accounting for specific characteristics of the wound site, the DNA vector and delivery method must be considered when assessing patient safety. In summary, studies that examine the use of specific delivery methods and DNA vectors in periodontal tissue engineering reflect the aim to maximize the duration of growth factor expression, optimize delivery method to periodontal defect, and minimize patient risk.

Recently, a combination of an AAV-delivered angiogenic molecule such as VEGF, BMP signaling receptor (caALK2), and RANKL (receptor activator of nuclear factor kappa B ligand) were demonstrated to promote bone allograft turnover and osteogenesis as a mode to enrich human bone allografts [112]. To date, combinations of VEGF/BMP [113] and PDGF/VEGF [95] have been performed with highly positive synergistic responses in bone repair. Promising preliminary results from preclinical studies reveal that host modulation achieved through gene delivery of soluble proteins, such as tumor necrosis factor receptor-1, reduces tumor necrosis factor activity and inhibits alveolar bone loss [101]. These results are comparable to the findings in the research on rheumatoid arthritis, in which pathogenesis, including high tumor necrosis factor activity and pathways for bone resorption, is similar [114].

Preclinical studies that evaluate growth factor gene therapy for tissue engineering

To overcome the short half-lives of growth factor peptides in vivo, gene therapy that uses a vector that encodes the growth factor is utilized to stimulate tissue regeneration. So far, two main strategies of gene vector delivery have been applied to periodontal tissue engineering. Gene vectors can be introduced directly to the target site (in vivo technique) [99], or selected cells can be harvested, expanded, genetically transduced, and then reimplanted (ex vivo technique) (Fig. 3) [98]. In vivo gene transfer involves the insertion of the gene of interest directly into the body anticipating the genetic modification of the target cell. Ex vivo gene transfer includes the incorporation of genetic material into cells exposed from a tissue biopsy with subsequent reimplantation into the recipient.

Platelet-derived growth factor gene delivery

The application of PDGF-gene transfer strategies to tissue engineering originally was generated to improve healing in soft tissue wounds, such as skin lesions [115]. Plasmid [116] and Ad/PDGF gene delivery [117] have been evaluated in preclinical and human trials. The latter approach has been able to exhibit more safety favorable for clinical use, however. [111].

Early studies in dental applications using recombinant adenoviral vectors that encode PDGF demonstrated the ability of these vector constructs to

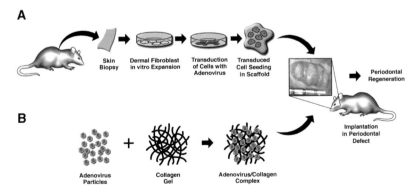

Fig. 3. Gene delivery approaches for periodontal tissue engineering. (*A*) Ex vivo gene delivery involves the harvesting of tissue biopsies, expansion of cell populations, genetic manipulations of cells, and subsequent transplantation to periodontal osseous defects. (*B*) The in vivo gene transfer approach involves the direct delivery of growth factor transgenes to the periodontal osseous defects.

transduce potently the cells isolated from the periodontium (eg, osteoblasts, cementoblasts, PDL cells, and gingival fibroblasts) [118,119]. These studies revealed the extensive and prolonged transduction of periodontal-derived cells. Chen and Giannobile [120] were able to demonstrate the prolonged effects of Ad delivery of PDGF for the better understanding of sustained PDGF signaling. An ex vivo investigation by Anusaksathien and colleagues [121] showed that the expression of PDGF genes was prolonged for up to 10 days in gingival wounds. Ad encoding PDGF-β transduced gingival fibroblasts and enhanced defect fill by induction of human gingival fibroblast migration and proliferation. On the other hand, continuous exposure of cementoblasts to PDGF-α had an inhibitory effect on cementum mineralization, possibly via the upregulation of osteopontin and subsequent enhancement of multinucleated giant cells in cementum-engineered scaffolds. Ad/PDGF-1308 (a dominant-negative mutant of PDGF) inhibited mineralization of tissue-engineered cementum possibly because of downregulation of bone sialoprotein and osteocalcin with a persistence of stimulation of multinucleated giant cells. These findings suggested that continuous exogenous delivery of PDGF-α may delay mineral formation induced by cementoblasts, whereas PDGF clearly is required for mineral neogenesis [122].

Jin and colleagues [99] demonstrated that direct in vivo gene transfer of PDGF-B stimulated tissue regeneration in large periodontal defects. Descriptive histology and histomorphometry revealed that human PDGF-B gene delivery promotes the regeneration of cementum and alveolar bone, whereas PDGF-1308, a dominant-negative mutant of PDGF-A, has minimal effects on periodontal tissue regeneration (Fig. 4).

Bone morphogenetic protein gene delivery

An experimental study in rodents by Lieberman and colleagues [123] demonstrated gene therapy for bone regeneration, with results revealing that the transduction of bone marrow stromal cells with rhBMP-2 lead to bone formation within an experimental defect comparable to skeletal bone. Another group was similarly able to regenerate skeletal bone by directly administering Ad5/BMP-2 into a bony segmental defect in rabbits [124]. Additional advances in the area of orthopedic gene therapy using viral delivery of BMP-2 have provided further evidence for the ability of in vivo and ex vivo bone engineering [125–128]. Franceschi and colleagues [100] investigated in vitro and in vivo Ad gene transfer of BMP-7 for bone formation. Ad-transduced nonosteogenic cells also were found to differentiate into bone-forming cells and produce BMP-7 [45] or BMP-2 [125] in vitro and in vivo. In another study by Huang and colleagues [129], plasmid DNA encoding for BMP-4 administered with a scaffold delivery system was found to enhance bone formation when compared with blank scaffolds.

In an early approach to regenerate alveolar bone in an animal model, the ex vivo delivery of Ad-encoding murine BMP-7 was found to promote periodontal tissue regeneration in large mandibular periodontal bone defects

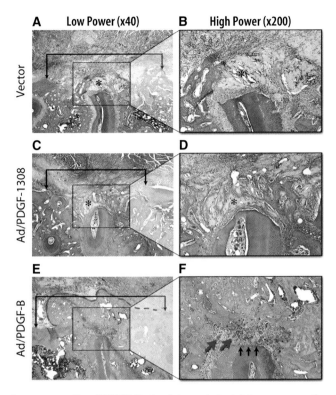

Fig. 4. In vivo gene transfer of PDGF-B stimulates periodontal tissue regeneration. Histologic microphotographs of periodontal alveolar bone defects treated for 14 days after gene delivery of Ad/PDGF-B, Ad/PDGF-1308, or vector alone. (*A, C, E*, original magnification ×40; *B, D, F*, original magnification ×200.) Brackets in the low-power (×40) slides indicate alveolar bone wound edges, with no significant differences between the sizes of the defects based on histomorphometric analyses. Limited alveolar bone formation occurred in the Ad/PDGF-1308 and vector alone defects, whereas significant bone bridging was noted most extensively in sites treated with Ad/PDGF-B (*red dashed line*). (*F*) A thin layer of newly formed cementum (*black arrows*) was observed only in the Ad/PDGF-B–treated defects. More vascularization (*blue arrows*) was seen in the periodontal ligament region of the Ad/PDGF-B–treated lesions. Asterisks indicate the collagen carrier. (*Adapted from* Jin Q, Anusaksathien O, Webb SA, et al. Engineering of tooth-supporting structures by delivery of PDGF gene therapy vectors. Mol Ther 2004;9(4):522; with permission.)

[98]. BMP-7 gene transfer not only enhanced alveolar bone repair but also stimulated cementogenesis and PDL fiber formation. Of interest, the alveolar bone formation was found to occur via a cartilage intermediate. When genes that encoded the BMP antagonist noggin were delivered, inhibition of periodontal tissue formation resulted [130]. A recent study by Dunn and colleagues [131] showed that direct in vivo gene delivery of Ad/BMP-7 in a collagen gel carrier promoted successful regeneration of alveolar bone defects around dental implants. These experiments provide promising

evidence that shows the feasibility of in vivo and ex vivo gene therapy for periodontal tissue regeneration and peri-implant osseointegration.

Future perspectives: targeted gene therapy in vivo

Major advances have been made over the past decade in the reconstruction of complex periodontal and alveolar bone wounds that have resulted from disease or injury. Developments in scaffolding matrices for cell, protein, and gene delivery have demonstrated significant potential to provide "smart" biomaterials that can interact with the matrix, cells, and bioactive factors. The targeting of signaling molecules or growth factors (via proteins or genes) to periodontia has led to significant new knowledge generation using factors that promote cell replication, differentiation, matrix biosynthesis, and angiogenesis. A major challenge that has been less studied is the modulation of the exuberant host response to microbial contamination that plagues the periodontal wound microenvironment. For improvements in the outcomes in periodontal regenerative medicine, scientists must examine dual delivery of host modifiers or anti-infective agents to optimize the results of therapy. Further advancements in the field will continue to rely heavily on multidisciplinary approaches that combine engineering, dentistry, medicine, and infectious disease specialists in repairing the complex periodontal wound environment.

Summary

This article highlights the active developments in the field of periodontal regenerative medicine. Significant advancements have been made within the areas of scaffold design to promote targeted delivery of cells, genes, and proteins to chronic periodontal wounds. Results from preclinical and early clinical studies are presented, with special emphasis on the use of growth factors to promote periodontal and peri-implant bone repair.

References

[1] Page RC, Offenbacher S, Schroeder HE, et al. Advances in the pathogenesis of periodontitis: summary of developments, clinical implications and future directions. J Periodontol Res 2000 1997;14:216–48.
[2] Williams RC. Periodontal disease. N Engl J Med 1990;322(6):373–82.
[3] Brown LJ, Loe H. Prevalence, extent, severity and progression of periodontal disease. Periodontology 2000 1993;2:57–71.
[4] Kocher T, Konig J, Dzierzon U, et al. Disease progression in periodontally treated and untreated patients: a retrospective study. J Clin Periodontol 2000;27(11):866–72.
[5] Heitz-Mayfield LJ, Schatzle M, Loe H, et al. Clinical course of chronic periodontitis. II. Incidence, characteristics and time of occurrence of the initial periodontal lesion. J Clin Periodontol 2003;30(10):902–8.

[6] Schatzle M, Loe H, Lang NP, et al. Clinical course of chronic periodontitis. III. Patterns, variations and risks of attachment loss. J Clin Periodontol 2003;30(10):909–18.

[7] Taba M Jr, Jin Q, Sugai JV, et al. Current concepts in periodontal bioengineering. Orthod Craniofac Res 2005;8(4):292–302.

[8] Gurinsky BS, Mills MP, Mellonig JT. Clinical evaluation of demineralized freeze-dried bone allograft and enamel matrix derivative versus enamel matrix derivative alone for the treatment of periodontal osseous defects in humans. J Periodontol 2004;75(10): 1309–18.

[9] Kimble KM, Eber RM, Soehren S, et al. Treatment of gingival recession using a collagen membrane with or without the use of demineralized freeze-dried bone allograft for space maintenance. J Periodontol 2004;75(2):210–20.

[10] Trejo PM, Weltman R, Caffesse R. Treatment of intraosseous defects with bioabsorbable barriers alone or in combination with decalcified freeze-dried bone allograft: a randomized clinical trial. J Periodontol 2000;71(12):1852–61.

[11] Hartman GA, Arnold RM, Mills MP, et al. Clinical and histologic evaluation of anorganic bovine bone collagen with or without a collagen barrier. Int J Periodontics Restorative Dent 2004;24(2):127–35.

[12] Camelo M, Nevins ML, Lynch SE, et al. Periodontal regeneration with an autogenous bone-Bio-Oss composite graft and a Bio-Gide membrane. Int J Periodontics Restorative Dent 2001;21(2):109–19.

[13] Mellonig JT. Human histologic evaluation of a bovine-derived bone xenograft in the treatment of periodontal osseous defects. Int J Periodontics Restorative Dent 2000; 20(1):19–29.

[14] Nevins ML, Camelo M, Nevins M, et al. Human histologic evaluation of bioactive ceramic in the treatment of periodontal osseous defects. Int J Periodontics Restorative Dent 2000; 20(5):458–67.

[15] Richardson CR, Mellonig JT, Brunsvold MA, et al. Clinical evaluation of Bio-Oss: a bovine-derived xenograft for the treatment of periodontal osseous defects in humans. J Clin Periodontol 1999;26(7):421–8.

[16] Palti A, Hoch T. A concept for the treatment of various dental bone defects. Implant Dent 2002;11(1):73–8.

[17] Scher EL, Day RB, Speight PM. New bone formation after a sinus lift procedure using demineralized freeze-dried bone and tricalcium phosphate. Implant Dent 1999;8(1):49–53.

[18] Nery EB, LeGeros RZ, Lynch KL, et al. Tissue response to biphasic calcium phosphate ceramic with different ratios of HA/beta TCP in periodontal osseous defects. J Periodontol 1992;63(9):729–35.

[19] Sculean A, Pietruska M, Schwarz F, et al. Healing of human intrabony defects following regenerative periodontal therapy with an enamel matrix protein derivative alone or combined with a bioactive glass: a controlled clinical study. J Clin Periodontol 2005;32(1): 111–7.

[20] Reynolds MA, Aichelmann-Reidy ME, Branch-Mays GL, et al. The efficacy of bone replacement grafts in the treatment of periodontal osseous defects: a systematic review. Ann Periodontol 2003;8(1):227–65.

[21] Trombelli L, Heitz-Mayfield LJ, Needleman I, et al. A systematic review of graft materials and biological agents for periodontal intraosseous defects. J Clin Periodontol 2002; 29(Suppl 3):117–35 [discussion 60–2].

[22] Fetner AE, Hartigan MS, Low SB. Periodontal repair using PerioGlas in nonhuman primates: clinical and histologic observations. Compendium 1994;15(7):932.

[23] Trombelli L, Minenna L, Farina R, et al. Guided tissue regeneration in human gingival recessions: a 10-year follow-up study. J Clin Periodontol 2005;32(1):16–20.

[24] Moses O, Pitaru S, Artzi Z, et al. Healing of dehiscence-type defects in implants placed together with different barrier membranes: a comparative clinical study. Clin Oral Implants Res 2005;16(2):210–9.

[25] Murphy KG, Gunsolley JC. Guided tissue regeneration for the treatment of periodontal intrabony and furcation defects: a systematic review. Ann Periodontol 2003;8(1):266–302.

[26] Needleman I, Tucker R, Giedrys-Leeper E, et al. A systematic review of guided tissue regeneration for periodontal infrabony defects. J Periodontal Res 2002;37(5):380–8.

[27] Minenna L, Herrero F, Sanz M, et al. Adjunctive effect of a polylactide/polyglycolide copolymer in the treatment of deep periodontal intra-osseous defects: a randomized clinical trial. J Clin Periodontol 2005;32(5):456–61.

[28] Stavropoulos A, Sculean A, Karring T. GTR treatment of intrabony defects with PLA/PGA copolymer or collagen bioresorbable membranes in combination with deproteinized bovine bone (Bio-Oss). Clin Oral Investig 2004;8(4):226–32.

[29] Parashis A, Andronikaki-Faldami A, Tsiklakis K. Clinical and radiographic comparison of three regenerative procedures in the treatment of intrabony defects. Int J Periodontics Restorative Dent 2004;24(1):81–90.

[30] Sculean A, Chiantella GC, Windisch P, et al. Healing of intra-bony defects following treatment with a composite bovine-derived xenograft (Bio-Oss Collagen) in combination with a collagen membrane (Bio-Gide PERIO). J Clin Periodontol 2005;32(7):720–4.

[31] Owczarek B, Kiernicka M, Galkowska E, et al. The application of Bio-Oss and Bio-Gide as implant materials in the complex treatment of aggressive periodontitis. Ann Univ Mariae Curie Sklodowska Med 2003;58(1):392–6.

[32] Camelo M, Nevins ML, Schenk RK, et al. Clinical, radiographic, and histologic evaluation of human periodontal defects treated with Bio-Oss and Bio-Gide. Int J Periodontics Restorative Dent 1998;18(4):321–31.

[33] Rasperini G, Silvestri M, Ricci G. Long-term clinical observation of treatment of infrabony defects with enamel matrix derivative (Emdogain): surgical reentry. Int J Periodontics Restorative Dent 2005;25(2):121–7.

[34] Rosing CK, Aass AM, Mavropoulos A, et al. Clinical and radiographic effects of enamel matrix derivative in the treatment of intrabony periodontal defects: a 12-month longitudinal placebo-controlled clinical trial in adult periodontitis patients. J Periodontol 2005;76(1):129–33.

[35] Sanz M, Tonetti MS, Zabalegui I, et al. Treatment of intrabony defects with enamel matrix proteins or barrier membranes: results from a multicenter practice-based clinical trial. J Periodontol 2004;75(5):726–33.

[36] Francetti L, Del Fabbro M, Basso M, et al. Enamel matrix proteins in the treatment of intra-bony defects: a prospective 24-month clinical trial. J Clin Periodontol 2004;31(1):52–9.

[37] Tonetti MS, Lang NP, Cortellini P, et al. Enamel matrix proteins in the regenerative therapy of deep intrabony defects. J Clin Periodontol 2002;29(4):317–25.

[38] McCulloch CA. Basic considerations in periodontal wound healing to achieve regeneration. J Periodontol 2000;1:16–25.

[39] Anusaksathien O, Giannobile WV. Growth factor delivery to re-engineer periodontal tissues. Curr Pharm Biotechnol 2002;3(2):129–39.

[40] Tozum TF, Demiralp B. Platelet-rich plasma: a promising innovation in dentistry. J Can Dent Assoc 2003;69(10):664.

[41] Okuda K, Kawase T, Momose M, et al. Platelet-rich plasma contains high levels of platelet-derived growth factor and transforming growth factor-beta and modulates the proliferation of periodontally related cells in vitro. J Periodontol 2003;74(6):849–57.

[42] Marcopoulou CE, Vavouraki HN, Dereka XE, et al. Proliferative effect of growth factors TGF-beta1, PDGF-BB and rhBMP-2 on human gingival fibroblasts and periodontal ligament cells. J Int Acad Periodontol 2003;5(3):63–70.

[43] Bosshardt DD. Are cementoblasts a subpopulation of osteoblasts or a unique phenotype? J Dent Res 2005;84(5):390–406.

[44] Sykaras N, Opperman LA. Bone morphogenetic proteins (BMPs): how do they function and what can they offer the clinician? J Oral Sci 2003;45(2):57–73.

[45] Krebsbach PH, Gu K, Franceschi RT, et al. Gene therapy-directed osteogenesis: BMP-7-transduced human fibroblasts form bone in vivo. Hum Gene Ther 2000;11(8): 1201–10.

[46] Giannobile WV. Periodontal tissue engineering by growth factors. Bone 1996;19(1 Suppl): 23S–37.

[47] Nakashima M, Reddi AH. The application of bone morphogenetic proteins to dental tissue engineering. Nat Biotechnol 2003;21(9):1025–32.

[48] Cochran DL, Wozney JM. Biological mediators for periodontal regeneration. J Periodontol 2000 1999;19:40–58.

[49] Rutherford RB, Niekrash CE, Kennedy JE, et al. Platelet-derived and insulin-like growth factors stimulate regeneration of periodontal attachment in monkeys. J Periodontal Res 1992;27(4 Pt 1):285–90.

[50] Giannobile WV, Finkelman RD, Lynch SE. Comparison of canine and non-human primate animal models for periodontal regenerative therapy: results following a single administration of PDGF/IGF-I. J Periodontol 1994;65(12):1158–68.

[51] Camelo M, Nevins ML, Schenk RK, et al. Periodontal regeneration in human Class II furcations using purified recombinant human platelet-derived growth factor-BB (rhPDGF-BB) with bone allograft. Int J Periodontics Restorative Dent 2003;23(3):213–25.

[52] Ojima Y, Mizuno M, Kuboki Y, et al. In vitro effect of platelet-derived growth factor-BB on collagen synthesis and proliferation of human periodontal ligament cells. Oral Dis 2003; 9(3):144–51.

[53] Nevins M, Giannobile WV, McGuire MK, et al. Platelet-derived growth factor (rhPDGF-BB) stimulates bone fill and rate of attachment level gain: results of a large multi-center randomized controlled trial. J Periodontol 2005;76(12):2205–15.

[54] Howell TH, Fiorellini JP, Paquette DW, et al. A phase I/II clinical trial to evaluate a combination of recombinant human platelet-derived growth factor-BB and recombinant human insulin-like growth factor-I in patients with periodontal disease. J Periodontol 1997; 68(12):1186–93.

[55] Lynch SE, de Castilla GR, Williams RC, et al. The effects of short-term application of a combination of platelet-derived and insulin-like growth factors on periodontal wound healing. J Periodontol 1991;62(7):458–67.

[56] Giannobile WV, Ryan S, Shih MS, et al. Recombinant human osteogenic protein-1 (OP-1) stimulates periodontal wound healing in class III furcation defects. J Periodontol 1998; 69(2):129–37.

[57] Murakami S, Takayama S, Kitamura M, et al. Recombinant human basic fibroblast growth factor (bFGF) stimulates periodontal regeneration in class II furcation defects created in beagle dogs. J Periodontal Res 2003;38(1):97–103.

[58] Sigurdsson TJ, Lee MB, Kubota K, et al. Periodontal repair in dogs: recombinant human bone morphogenetic protein-2 significantly enhances periodontal regeneration. J Periodontol 1995;66(2):131–8.

[59] Takayama S, Murakami S, Shimabukuro Y, et al. Periodontal regeneration by FGF-2 (bFGF) in primate models. J Dent Res 2001;80(12):2075–9.

[60] Terranova VP, Odziemiec C, Tweden KS, et al. Repopulation of dentin surfaces by periodontal ligament cells and endothelial cells: effect of basic fibroblast growth factor. J Periodontol 1989;60(6):293–301.

[61] Huang KK, Shen C, Chiang CY, et al. Effects of bone morphogenetic protein-6 on periodontal wound healing in a fenestration defect of rats. J Periodontal Res 2005;40(1): 1–10.

[62] Wikesjo UM, Qahash M, Thomson RC, et al. rhBMP-2 significantly enhances guided bone regeneration. Clin Oral Implants Res 2004;15(2):194–204.

[63] Wikesjo UM, Sorensen RG, Kinoshita A, et al. Periodontal repair in dogs: effect of recombinant human bone morphogenetic protein-12 (rhBMP-12) on regeneration of alveolar bone and periodontal attachment. J Clin Periodontol 2004;31(8):662–70.

[64] Sorensen RG, Wikesjo UM, Kinoshita A, et al. Periodontal repair in dogs: evaluation of a bioresorbable calcium phosphate cement (Ceredex) as a carrier for rhBMP-2. J Clin Periodontol 2004;31(9):796–804.

[65] Gao Y, Yang L, Fang YR, et al. The inductive effect of bone morphogenetic protein (BMP) on human periodontal fibroblast-like cells in vitro. J Osaka Dent Univ 1995;29(1):9–17.

[66] Jung RE, Glauser R, Scharer P, et al. Effect of rhBMP-2 on guided bone regeneration in humans. Clin Oral Implants Res 2003;14(5):556–68.

[67] Meraw SJ, Reeve CM, Lohse CM, et al. Treatment of peri-implant defects with combination growth factor cement. J Periodontol 2000;71(1):8–13.

[68] Heldin P, Laurent TC, Heldin CH. Effect of growth factors on hyaluronan synthesis in cultured human fibroblasts. Biochem J 1989;258(3):919–22.

[69] Kaplan DR, Chao FC, Stiles CD, et al. Platelet alpha granules contain a growth factor for fibroblasts. Blood 1979;53(6):1043–52.

[70] Rosenkranz S, Kazlauskas A. Evidence for distinct signaling properties and biological responses induced by the PDGF receptor alpha and beta subtypes. Growth Factors 1999; 16(3):201–16.

[71] Seppa H, Grotendorst G, Seppa S, et al. Platelet-derived growth factor in chemotactic for fibroblasts. J Cell Biol 1982;92(2):584–8.

[72] Parkar MH, Kuru L, Giouzeli M, et al. Expression of growth-factor receptors in normal and regenerating human periodontal cells. Arch Oral Biol 2001;46(3):275–84.

[73] Nishimura F, Terranova VP. Comparative study of the chemotactic responses of periodontal ligament cells and gingival fibroblasts to polypeptide growth factors. J Dent Res 1996; 75(4):986–92.

[74] Oates TW, Rouse CA, Cochran DL. Mitogenic effects of growth factors on human periodontal ligament cells in vitro. J Periodontol 1993;64(2):142–8.

[75] Haase HR, Clarkson RW, Waters MJ, et al. Growth factor modulation of mitogenic responses and proteoglycan synthesis by human periodontal fibroblasts. J Cell Physiol 1998;174(3):353–61.

[76] Zaman KU, Sugaya T, Kato H. Effect of recombinant human platelet-derived growth factor-BB and bone morphogenetic protein-2 application to demineralized dentin on early periodontal ligament cell response. J Periodontal Res 1999;34(5):244–50.

[77] Giannobile WV, Hernandez RA, Finkelman RD, et al. Comparative effects of platelet-derived growth factor-BB and insulin-like growth factor-I, individually and in combination, on periodontal regeneration in *Macaca fascicularis*. J Periodontal Res 1996;31(5):301–12.

[78] Lynch SE, Williams RC, Polson AM, et al. A combination of platelet-derived and insulin-like growth factors enhances periodontal regeneration. J Clin Periodontol 1989;16(8): 545–8.

[79] Matsuda N, Lin WL, Kumar NM, et al. Mitogenic, chemotactic, and synthetic responses of rat periodontal ligament fibroblastic cells to polypeptide growth factors in vitro. J Periodontol 1992;63(6):515–25.

[80] Wozney JM, Rosen V, Celeste AJ, et al. Novel regulators of bone formation: molecular clones and activities. Science 1988;242(4885):1528–34.

[81] Reddi AH. Role of morphogenetic proteins in skeletal tissue engineering and regeneration. Nat Biotechnol 1998;16(3):247–52.

[82] Urist MR. Bone: formation by autoinduction. Science 1965;150(698):893–9.

[83] Reddi AH. Bone morphogenetic proteins: from basic science to clinical applications. J Bone Joint Surg Am 2001;83A(Suppl 1):S1–6.

[84] Aberg T, Wozney J, Thesleff I. Expression patterns of bone morphogenetic proteins (BMPs) in the developing mouse tooth suggest roles in morphogenesis and cell differentiation. Dev Dyn 1997;210(4):383–96.

[85] Amar S, Chung KM, Nam SH, et al. Markers of bone and cementum formation accumulate in tissues regenerated in periodontal defects treated with expanded polytetrafluoroethylene membranes. J Periodontal Res 1997;32(1 Pt 2):148–58.

[86] Lutolf MP, Weber FE, Schmoekel HG, et al. Repair of bone defects using synthetic mimetics of collagenous extracellular matrices. Nat Biotechnol 2003;21(5):513–8.

[87] Wikesjo UM, Xiropaidis AV, Thomson RC, et al. Periodontal repair in dogs: rhBMP-2 significantly enhances bone formation under provisions for guided tissue regeneration. J Clin Periodontol 2003;30(8):705–14.

[88] Fiorellini JP, Howell TH, Cochran D, et al. Randomized study evaluating recombinant human bone morphogenetic protein-2 for extraction socket augmentation. J Periodontol 2005;76(4):605–13.

[89] Rutherford RB, Sampath TK, Rueger DC, et al. Use of bovine osteogenic protein to promote rapid osseointegration of endosseous dental implants. Int J Oral Maxillofac Implants 1992;7(3):297–301.

[90] van den Bergh JP, ten Bruggenkate CM, Groeneveld HH, et al. Recombinant human bone morphogenetic protein-7 in maxillary sinus floor elevation surgery in 3 patients compared to autogenous bone grafts: a clinical pilot study. J Clin Periodontol 2000; 27(9):627–36.

[91] Anusaksathien O, Jin Q, Ma PX, et al. Scaffolding in periodontal engineering. In: Ma PX, Eliseeff J, editors. Scaffolding in tissue engineering. Boca Raton (FL): CRC Press; 2005. p. 427–44.

[92] Lutolf MP, Hubbell JA. Synthetic biomaterials as instructive extracellular microenvironments for morphogenesis in tissue engineering. Nat Biotechnol 2005;23(1):47–55.

[93] Babensee JE, McIntire LV, Mikos AG. Growth factor delivery for tissue engineering. Pharm Res 2000;17(5):497–504.

[94] Hutmacher DW, Teoh SH, Zein I, et al. Tissue engineering research: the engineer's role. Med Device Technol 2000;11(1):33–9.

[95] Richardson TP, Peters MC, Ennett AB, et al. Polymeric system for dual growth factor delivery. Nat Biotechnol 2001;19(11):1029–34.

[96] Baum BJ, Goldsmith CM, Kok MR, et al. Advances in vector-mediated gene transfer. Immunol Lett 2003;90(2–3):145–9.

[97] Giannobile WV. What does the future hold for periodontal tissue engineering? Int J Periodontics Restorative Dent 2002;22(1):6–7.

[98] Jin QM, Anusaksathien O, Webb SA, et al. Gene therapy of bone morphogenetic protein for periodontal tissue engineering. J Periodontol 2003;74(2):202–13.

[99] Jin Q, Anusaksathien O, Webb SA, et al. Engineering of tooth-supporting structures by delivery of PDGF gene therapy vectors. Mol Ther 2004;9(4):519–26.

[100] Franceschi RT, Wang D, Krebsbach PH, et al. Gene therapy for bone formation: in vitro and in vivo osteogenic activity of an adenovirus expressing BMP7. J Cell Biochem 2000; 78(3):476–86.

[101] Taba M Jr, Huffer HH, Shelburne CE, et al. Gene delivery of TNFR:Fc by adeno-associated virus vector blocks progression of periodontitis [abstract 677]. In: Programs and abstracts of the American Society of Gene Therapy's Eighth Annual Meeting. Saint Louis (MO): American Society of Gene Therapy; 2005. p. 262.

[102] Friedmann T. The maturation of human gene therapy. Acta Paediatr 1996;85(11):1261–5.

[103] Baum BJ, Kok M, Tran SD, et al. The impact of gene therapy on dentistry: a revisiting after six years. J Am Dent Assoc 2002;133(1):35–44.

[104] Baum BJ, O'Connell BC. The impact of gene therapy on dentistry. J Am Dent Assoc 1995; 126(2):179–89.

[105] Parekh-Olmedo H, Ferrara L, Brachman E, et al. Gene therapy progress and prospects: targeted gene repair. Gene Ther 2005;12(8):639–46.

[106] Muramatsu S, Tsukada H, Nakano I, et al. Gene therapy for Parkinson's disease using recombinant adeno-associated viral vectors. Expert Opin Biol Ther 2005;5(5): 663–71.

[107] Partridge KA, Oreffo RO. Gene delivery in bone tissue engineering: progress and prospects using viral and nonviral strategies. Tissue Eng 2004;10(1–2):295–307.

[108] Worgall S. A realistic chance for gene therapy in the near future. Pediatr Nephrol 2005;
      20(2):118–24.
[109] Zolotukhin S. Production of recombinant adeno-associated virus vectors. Hum Gene Ther
      2005;16(5):551–7.
[110] Sirninger J, Muller C, Braag S, et al. Functional characterization of a recombinant adeno-
      associated virus 5-pseudotyped cystic fibrosis transmembrane conductance regulator vec-
      tor. Hum Gene Ther 2004;15(9):832–41.
[111] Gu DL, Nguyen T, Gonzalez AM, et al. Adenovirus encoding human platelet-derived
      growth factor-B delivered in collagen exhibits safety, biodistribution, and immunogenicity
      profiles favorable for clinical use. Mol Ther 2004;9(5):699–711.
[112] Ito H, Koefoed M, Tiyapatanaputi P, et al. Remodeling of cortical bone allografts mediated
      by adherent rAAV-RANKL and VEGF gene therapy. Nat Med 2005;11(3):291–7.
[113] Peng H, Wright V, Usas A, et al. Synergistic enhancement of bone formation and healing by
      stem cell-expressed VEGF and bone morphogenetic protein-4. J Clin Invest 2002;110(6):
      751–9.
[114] Ramamurthy NS, Greenwald RA, Celiker MY, et al. Experimental arthritis in rats induces
      biomarkers of periodontitis which are ameliorated by gene therapy with tissue inhibitor of
      matrix metalloproteinases. J Periodontol 2005;76(2):229–33.
[115] Crombleholme TM. Adenoviral-mediated gene transfer in wound healing. Wound Repair
      Regen 2000;8(6):460–72.
[116] Hijjawi J, Mogford JE, Chandler LA, et al. Platelet-derived growth factor B, but not fibro-
      blast growth factor 2, plasmid DNA improves survival of ischemic mucocutaneous flaps.
      Arch Surg 2004;139(2):142–7.
[117] Printz MA, Gonzalez AM, Cunningham M, et al. Fibroblast growth factor 2-retargeted ad-
      enoviral vectors exhibit a modified biolocalization pattern and display reduced toxicity rel-
      ative to native adenoviral vectors. Hum Gene Ther 2000;11(1):191–204.
[118] Zhu Z, Lee CS, Tejeda KM, et al. Gene transfer and expression of platelet-derived growth
      factors modulate periodontal cellular activity. J Dent Res 2001;80(3):892–7.
[119] Giannobile WV, Lee CS, Tomala MP, et al. Platelet-derived growth factor (PDGF) gene
      delivery for application in periodontal tissue engineering. J Periodontol 2001;72(6):815–23.
[120] Chen QP, Giannobile WV. Adenoviral gene transfer of PDGF downregulates gas gene
      product PDGFalphaR and prolongs ERK and Akt/PKB activation. Am J Physiol Cell
      Physiol 2002;282(3):C538–44.
[121] Anusaksathien O, Webb SA, Jin QM, et al. Platelet-derived growth factor gene delivery
      stimulates ex vivo gingival repair. Tissue Eng 2003;9(4):745–56.
[122] Anusaksathien O, Jin Q, Zhao M, et al. Effect of sustained gene delivery of platelet-derived
      growth factor or its antagonist (PDGF-1308) on tissue-engineered cementum. J Periodon-
      tol 2004;75(3):429–40.
[123] Lieberman JR, Daluiski A, Stevenson S, et al. The effect of regional gene therapy with bone
      morphogenetic protein-2-producing bone-marrow cells on the repair of segmental femoral
      defects in rats. J Bone Joint Surg Am 1999;81(7):905–17.
[124] Baltzer AW, Lattermann C, Whalen JD, et al. Genetic enhancement of fracture repair: heal-
      ing of an experimental segmental defect by adenoviral transfer of the BMP-2 gene. Gene
      Ther 2000;7(9):734–9.
[125] Cheng SL, Lou J, Wright NM, et al. In vitro and in vivo induction of bone formation using
      a recombinant adenoviral vector carrying the human BMP-2 gene. Calcif Tissue Int 2001;
      68(2):87–94.
[126] Lee JY, Musgrave D, Pelinkovic D, et al. Effect of bone morphogenetic protein-2-express-
      ing muscle-derived cells on healing of critical-sized bone defects in mice. J Bone Joint Surg
      Am 2001;83A(7):1032–9.
[127] Lee JY, Peng H, Usas A, et al. Enhancement of bone healing based on ex vivo gene therapy
      using human muscle-derived cells expressing bone morphogenetic protein 2. Hum Gene
      Ther 2002;13(10):1201–11.

[128] Musgrave DS, Bosch P, Ghivizzani S, et al. Adenovirus-mediated direct gene therapy with bone morphogenetic protein-2 produces bone. Bone 1999;24(6):541–7.
[129] Huang YC, Simmons C, Kaigler D, et al. Bone regeneration in a rat cranial defect with delivery of PEI-condensed plasmid DNA encoding for bone morphogenetic protein-4 (BMP-4). Gene Ther 2005;12(5):418–26.
[130] Jin QM, Zhao M, Economides AN, et al. Noggin gene delivery inhibits cementoblast-induced mineralization. Connect Tissue Res 2004;45(1):50–9.
[131] Dunn CA, Jin Q, Taba M Jr, et al. BMP gene delivery for alveolar bone engineering at dental implant defects. Mol Ther 2005;11(2):294–9.

THE DENTAL
CLINICS
OF NORTH AMERICA

Dent Clin N Am 50 (2006) 265–276

A Review of New Developments in Tissue Engineering Therapy for Periodontitis

Taka Nakahara, DDS, PhD

*Section of Developmental and Regenerative Dentistry, School of Life Dentistry at Tokyo,
The Nippon Dental University, 1-9-20 Fujimi, Chiyoda-ku, Tokyo 102-8159, Japan*

Periodontitis is a highly prevalent chronic inflammatory disease and has been linked to systemic diseases, such as diabetes, cardiovascular disease, and respiratory diseases [1]. If untreated, this disorder can destroy the tissues that support the teeth (that is, the alveolar bone, periodontal ligament, cementum, and gingival tissue), which eventually leads to tooth loss. According to a survey performed in 1999 [2], roughly 50% of Japanese individuals in their 30s had lost at least one tooth, and the number of teeth lost per person increased sharply after the age of 40. Furthermore, more than 50% of Japanese people aged 85 years or more were found to be completely edentulous—that is, they had none of their 28 original teeth. Scaling and root planing are effective methods for preventing the progression of periodontitis in most cases. However, although these conventional treatments can eliminate the causes of periodontitis, they are unable to regenerate lost tissues, such as the alveolar bone, cementum, and periodontal ligament. In Japan, it is known that more than 80% of adults aged over 30 years have periodontal diseases, including gingivitis and periodontitis [2]. Thus, an urgent need exists to establish a new therapeutic method for this disease.

In 1993, Langer and colleagues [3] proposed tissue engineering as a possible technique for regenerating lost tissue, and the restoration of various human tissues and organs is starting to become a reality. The concept of tissue engineering was introduced originally to address the chronic shortage of donated organs. This approach reconstructs natural target tissue by combining three elements: a scaffold or matrix, signaling molecules (for example, growth and differentiation factors and genes), and cells. Current approaches

This work was supported by a Grant-in-Aid for Scientific Research 16791322 from the Ministry of Education, Culture, Sports, Science, and Technology of Japan.

E-mail address: t.nakahara@tky.ndu.ac.jp

0011-8532/06/$ - see front matter. Published by Elsevier Inc.
doi:10.1016/j.cden.2005.11.004

to tissue engineering can be divided roughly into two main types: ex vivo and in vivo (Fig. 1). In the former, the target tissue is created in a laboratory by culturing cells on biodegradable scaffolds in the presence of specific trophic factors before their transplantation into the body [4,5]. In the latter approach, the three elements mentioned above are placed into a tissue defect "in situ," and the tissue is restored by maximizing the natural healing capacity of the body by creating a local environment that is favorable for regeneration [6–8].

This article reviews tissue regeneration techniques, with an emphasis on the restoration of periodontal tissues, and discusses possible future directions based on recent technologic advances.

Tissue engineering for periodontal tissue regeneration

Protein-based approaches

Growth and differentiation factors can regulate the adhesion, migration, proliferation, and differentiation of various types of cell by binding to appropriate receptors. Recent advances in genetic engineering technology have made it possible to obtain large quantities of human recombinant proteins. The use of growth and differentiation factors is the most popular tissue engineering approach for regenerating periodontal tissues. So far, several growth factors—including transforming growth factor-β (TGF-β) superfamily members, such as bone morphogenetic protein-2 (BMP-2), BMP-6, BMP-7, BMP-12, TGF-β, basic fibroblast growth factor (bFGF), and platelet-derived growth factor (PDGF)—have been used to regenerate periodontal tissues [9–16]. Moreover, studies are underway currently to test the clinical potential of some of these factors [15,16].

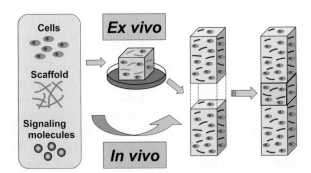

Fig. 1. Schematic representation of two major approaches to tissue engineering. First technique is to create tissue or organs in culture room by combining three elements (scaffold or matrix, signaling molecules, and cells) before transplanting tissue-engineered organ into patients (ex vivo approach). Second technique is to induce intrinsic healing activity at site of tissue defect using these three elements (in vivo approach).

Platelet-rich plasma (PRP) contains several platelet-released growth factors, including PDGF and TGF-β. PRP therefore represents an autologous growth factor cocktail that can be harvested from patients with minimal invasiveness and used for applications in oral and maxillofacial surgery [17–21]. PRP stimulates the proliferation of human osteogenic cells [22,23] and periodontal ligament cells [24]. However, the benefits of this approach remain controversial: although some investigators have reported positive effects on bone formation [17–19], others have failed to detect any improvement [20,21]. This discrepancy in wound-healing outcomes might be explained partly by interindividual variation because PRP is an autologous resource. Moreover, the optimal concentrations of the calcium and thrombin, which are the inducers of platelet activation leading to growth factor release, are unclear [25]. To maximize the healing potential of the application of PRP to bone regeneration, it is necessary to introduce sufficient number of osteogenic stem cells that respond to PRP-derived growth factors by way of autologous bone grafts or the implantation of a cell-scaffold construct [17]. If such a cell source and scaffold can be supplied at the site of the defect, it has been shown by case studies to induce bone formation successfully [17–19]. Further information obtained from basic research at the cellular and molecular level could help this to become a reliable technique for assisting wound healing. The combination of a drug delivery system (DDS) with PRP may be effective, as the following paragraph shows.

The development of synthetic or natural polymer-delivery vehicles for the sustained release of growth and differentiation factors will be crucial for their clinical utility [26,27]. Locally-applied growth factors are defused away rapidly from the implantation site and have a short half-life as a result of a combination of physical and biologic degradation mechanisms. DDS using biomaterial vehicles has allowed the tissue-exposure time to be extended and protein stability to be maintained within the body. Nakahara and colleagues [28,29] investigated the effectiveness of a tissue regeneration device combining a collagen sponge-scaffold material and gelatin microspheres, which prolonged the period of bFGF release in beagles with artificially prepared intrabony periodontal defects. This report was the first to demonstrate the usefulness of DDS and cell scaffolds for targeted periodontal regeneration using a full-scale animal experimental model. In this controlled delivery system, positively charged bFGF molecules formed an ionic complex with acidic gelatin and were released gradually as a result of the degradation of the vehicle in vivo over an extended period. In the bFGF-treated group, 4 weeks after implantation, numerous capillary vessels were observed within the regenerated tissue around the residual gelatin vehicles containing bFGF. This observation indicated that the powerful angiogenic activity of bFGF still was present at this stage. These findings imply that a rich vascular supply is essential throughout the healing process to facilitate periodontal regeneration.

Currently, most delivery approaches involve a single growth factor. These techniques might be unable therefore to induce well-developed vascular networks leading to tissue regeneration, as angiogenesis results from a complicated series of cellular and molecular interactions. However, recent advances in polymeric technologies have allowed the delivery of multiple angiogenic growth factors with distinct kinetics by a single scaffold. For example, Richardson and colleagues [30] reported the development of a new porous polymer scaffold that can deliver vascular endothelial growth factor (VEGF) and PDGF-BB. In this system, VEGF, which stimulates the outgrowth of immature vessels consisting of naked endothelial cells, is mixed with the polymer scaffold, resulting in its rapid release from the vehicle during the first days or weeks after implantation. Meanwhile, PDGF-BB, which stimulates the maturation and stabilization of nascent vessels by way of the recruitment of smooth-muscle cells, is pre-encapsulated within microspheres in the polymer scaffold, from which it is released by degradation in a delayed fashion. The controlled delivery of VEGF and PDGF-BB significantly increases the maturity of the resultant vessel networks. Similarly, Cao and colleagues [31] reported that a combination of PDGF-BB and FGF-2 synergistically induced stable vascular networks, whereas single growth factors were unable to maintain the newly formed blood vessels. Such dual growth factor-delivery technologies could be useful in periodontal tissue engineering.

Cell-based approaches

Cell transplantation is currently a hot topic in the medical field and cell-based therapy using autologous cells is expected to play a central clinical role in the future [32–34]. Several preclinical studies using mesenchymal stem cells (MSCs) have shown efficient reconstruction of bone defects larger than those that would spontaneously heal (that is, critical size defects) [35,36]. Dental cell-seeding studies have attempted to regenerate periodontal tissues since the 1990s [37–41], although clinical applications have become realistic only in recent years.

Kawaguchi and colleagues [42] used bone-marrow-derived MSCs in combination with atelocollagen to regenerate periodontal tissues in experimental class III furcation defects in dogs. After cell expansion for 2 weeks, autologous MSCs mixed with collagen gel were transplanted into the defects. In the MSC-treated groups, significant periodontal tissue structures were observed 1 month after implantation compared with the collagen gel group. However, at the experimental cell concentrations (2×10^6–10^7), no significant difference was observed between the extent of regeneration of the bone and cementum tissues. The investigators concluded that additional studies using different scaffold materials and a various range of cell concentrations would be required to obtain conclusive results. Akizuki and colleagues [43] used autologous periodontal ligament cells obtained from extracted tooth roots to fabricate cell sheets using a temperature-responsive cell-culture approach based on cell-sheet engineering. A special culture dish, in which the dish surface is hydrophobic under normal culture conditions at 37°C, allowing cells to attach themselves to it and grow but becomes hydrophilic at 20°C so that cells detach themselves spontaneously, was used [44]. This process enabled the collection of the confluent cell cultures as a single sheet in which the deposited extracellular matrix and cell-cell junction proteins remained intact, in contrast to traditional enzymatic treatments for cell detachment, which damage the cultured cells. Autologous periodontal ligament-cell sheets along with a reinforced hyaluronic-acid carrier were implanted into experimental dehiscence defects in dog molars. After 8 weeks, significantly improved periodontal tissue regeneration was observed compared with control cases that received the hyaluronic-acid cell carrier alone. Although further studies are needed to confirm the reproducibility of these regenerative effects, cell-sheet engineering has shown great potential as a new cell-based periodontal therapy.

Cell transplantation has been shown to promote periodontal regeneration compared with the carrier alone as the control. However, it remains unclear whether the transplanted cells differentiate into osteoblasts, cementoblasts, and fibroblasts—to form bone, cementum, and periodontal ligament, respectively—or whether they recruit surrounding host cells to facilitate the regeneration of the periodontal tissues. The fate of the transplanted cells can be determined by labeling them and, thereby, the localization of the transplanted cells within the regenerated tissue can be detected [45].

Cells that are harvested from patients are often frozen and stored for long periods before use in the treatment of periodontitis. Previous studies have demonstrated that cells that have been subjected to freezing and thawing retain the ability to form periodontal tissues, thereby confirming the usefulness of such autologous cells [40–42]. Stem cells are believed to be present in all organs of the body where they maintain tissue homeostasis. The existence of periodontal ligament stem cells (PDLSCs) has been debated for some time. However, one recent study obtained a PDLSC population from the periodontal ligament of human adult impacted third molars [46]. Hence, autologous cells, including PDLSCs, represent valuable patient-derived therapeutic resources for use in the natural reconstruction of tissue destroyed by periodontal diseases.

Gene delivery-based approaches

Numerous tissue regeneration studies have investigated various gene-delivery techniques [47–49]. These techniques involve a gene encoding a therapeutic protein being introduced into cells, which can then express the target protein. This technique avoids the problems associated with the protein-delivery method by maintaining constant protein levels at the site of the defect. Genetic engineering approaches generally consist of two modalities: in vivo and ex vivo gene delivery. In the former, gene constructs, such as expression plasmid DNA or a viral particle, are physically entrapped within a scaffold or matrix. When the scaffold containing the gene constructs is implanted into the tissue defect, the host cells migrate into the implant, take up the gene constructs and start to produce the encoded protein. By contrast, in the latter approach, cultured cells are transfected (in nonviral delivery systems) or transduced (in viral delivery systems) with gene constructs in vitro before they are transplanted into the tissue defect.

Jin and colleagues [50,51] investigated gene therapy by incorporating BMP-7 and PDGF-B genes into adenovirus vectors. Rat syngeneic dermal fibroblasts were transduced ex vivo with adenoviruses encoding BMP-7 (Ad-BMP-7). These cells were then seeded onto gelatin sponges and placed into periodontal osseous defects [50]. Ad-PDGF-B was used for in vivo direct gene transfer. This vector was initially mixed with a collagen matrix before implantation into rat periodontal alveolar bone defects [51]. These adenoviral gene-transfer approaches stimulated regenerative activities in the periodontal tissues, including osteogenesis, cementogenesis, and periodontal ligament formation. Moreover, in each experiment, minimal periodontal tissue regeneration was induced using Ad-noggin, which is an inhibitor of several BMPs [50], or Ad-PDGF-1308, which inhibits the effects of PDGF activity [51]. Thus, the usefulness of gene therapy for periodontitis has been documented in rats. However, it still remains necessary to confirm the safety and predictability of tissue regeneration that is induced by adenovirus vectors.

Although viral delivery systems have been used successfully in a broad range of tissues, they have some disadvantages, including the risks for mutagenesis, carcinogenesis, and invoking immune reactions in response to viral infection or viral proteins. The development of safer nonviral alternatives is now progressing. Bonadio and colleagues [52] reported that plasmid DNA encoding an active fragment of the human parathyroid hormone physically entrapped within a collagen matrix to form a moldable three-dimensional porous sponge could be used in bone tissue engineering applications. Cells recruited by the repair process took up the plasmid DNA within the collagen matrix and expressed the protein in vivo, which resulted in the generation of bone tissue. Bonadio and colleagues [52] demonstrated the potential utility of this nonviral gene delivery system in critical-size canine skeletal defects.

In a recent study, the sonic hedgehog (Shh) gene, which encodes an essential regulator protein of embryonic osteogenesis and the repair of bone fractures, was transduced into periosteal and fat-derived stem cells, and gingival fibroblasts, to regenerate rabbit cranial bone defects in an alginate and collagen matrix [53]. At 12 weeks postimplantation, a significant increase in bone regeneration was observed in all three Shh-transduced groups compared with the control. This study suggested that the modified cells coordinated the expression of multiple growth factors, such as the BMPs, implicated in bone formation, and demonstrated the potential use of such a novel gene-enhanced tissue engineering approach in bone regeneration.

In summary, gene delivery-based therapy focused on the regeneration of periodontal and osseous defects has been successful at the experimental level. These findings will encourage the further development of safe and reproducible tissue engineering approaches for clinical application.

Fig. 2 summarizes the tissue engineering approach for the activation of stem cells with the aim of tissue regeneration. Growth factors that are delivered to a local site bind to cell-surface receptors and send intracellular signals. Subsequently, the cells proliferate and differentiate. In addition, gene-transfer techniques might allow the delivery of therapeutic growth factors by way of genetically modified cells, leading to the sustained expression and release of target proteins to the surrounding tissues in vivo, which will further enhance the regenerative potential of stem cells.

Remarks and future directions

Which is more important target for tissue engineering, teeth or the tissues supporting them? In previous decades, numerous studies have investigated the regeneration of periodontal tissues as introduced in the present review. Recently, the focus has shifted, with two studies attempting to regenerate teeth [54,55]. However, although these groups successfully reconstituted the individual structural elements that make up a tooth crown (that is, the dentin, enamel, and dental pulp), neither managed to regulate the morphogenesis of the crown or to regenerate the tooth root. Further improvements

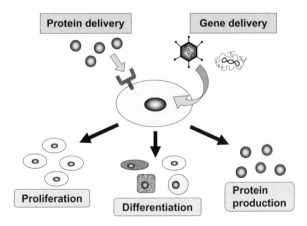

Fig. 2. Schematic representation of activation of stem cells through tissue-engineering approaches. Locally applied therapeutic proteins bind to appropriate receptors displayed at cell surface. Subsequently, cells are activated and undergo proliferation or differentiation. After taking up gene constructs through in vivo or ex vivo gene transfer using a plasmid or viral vector, genetically modified cells can either be seeded or migrate into scaffold, where they continuously secrete transgene-encoded therapeutic proteins into surrounding tissues.

and innovative approaches will be required to reconstruct "complete" teeth using tissue engineering.

Despite the recent interest in tooth regeneration, the view remains that, in a clinical setting, the fundamental goal is actually the regeneration of periodontal tissues, particularly centering on the periodontal ligament. If the periodontal ligament could be regenerated, an artificial tooth implant would suffice, yielding almost natural occlusion and mastication accompanied by real sensation while chewing. It is difficult to judge which theory is correct, but talking to patients about realizing the dream of regenerating teeth has revealed the huge impact that such technology would have on many of their lives. By extension, patient demand clearly defines the ultimate goals for the development of advanced regenerative dental techniques. Thus, the regeneration of teeth is likely to propose an important research topic, which is intimately related to the natural reconstruction of periodontium.

Guided tissue regeneration (GTR) was clinically applied in dental regenerative therapy before any other medical field, and the enamel matrix derivative, Emdogain, is the first periodontal therapy based on a biologic approach. These techniques are examples of first-generation regenerative therapies. The various attempts at tissue regeneration, which come under the general heading of "tissue engineering," introduced in the present review should probably be classed as "second-generation" regenerative medicine. This second-generation approach is making surprisingly rapid progress and its remit has expanded from its original application in the medical field to various related disciplines in which the introduction of biologic and engineering knowledge and skills are allowing the development of new approaches.

In the near future, third-generation periodontal therapies will involve nanoscale science [56–59] and moldless manufacturing technology commonly known as rapid prototyping (RP) [60] or solid free-form fabrication (SFF) [61]. These scientific and technologic innovations will make it possible to fabricate complex scaffolds that mimic the different structures and physiologic functions of natural fibro-osseous tissues, including those, such as periodontium, which consist of hard and soft tissues. The advancement of such technology might also make it possible to produce patient-specific cell-scaffold constructs with optimal distribution of cells and high vascular permeability [62,63].

In the context of regenerative dentistry, the various stem cells existing in human dental tissues are being isolated continuously from adult dental pulp [64], exfoliated deciduous teeth [65], and periodontal ligament [46]. The understanding of the molecular mechanisms that control stem cell function has been improving, although the translational research necessary to apply this knowledge to regenerative medicine is still in its infancy. Future studies will require the collaboration of researchers from different disciplines, including stem cell biology, material science, and of course, basic and clinical dentistry [66–68].

Conventional dental treatment has relied on symptomatic treatment and prosthetic restoration using artificial materials, and clinicians have tended to concentrate on improving their skills rather than developing new modes of treatment. To accelerate the clinical application of newly developed periodontal therapy, the important issues should be addressed while developing the periodontal therapeutic techniques. The ideal system for clinical use will be a simple procedure that provides one-step delivery of the gene/protein of interest with minimal manipulation. The development of such a therapeutic approach will enable wider clinical application that will benefit the increasing numbers of the aging population suffering from periodontitis.

References

[1] Amar S, Han X. The impact of periodontal infection on systemic diseases. Med Sci Monit 2003;9(12):RA291–9.
[2] Health Policy Bureau, Ministry of Health, Labour and Welfare. Report on the survey of dental diseases, 1999. Tokyo: Oral Health Association of Japan; 2001.
[3] Langer R, Vacanti JP. Tissue engineering. Science 1993;260(5110):920–6.
[4] Stock UA, Vacanti JP. Tissue engineering: current state and prospects. Annu Rev Med 2001; 52:443–51.
[5] Shieh SJ, Vacanti JP. State-of-the-art tissue engineering: from tissue engineering to organ building. Surgery 2005;137(1):1–7.
[6] Ikada Y. Tissue engineering research trends at Kyoto University. In: Ikada Y, editor. Tissue engineering for therapeutic use 1. Tokyo: Elsevier; 1998. p. 1–14.
[7] Shimizu Y. Tissue engineering for soft tissues. In: Ikada Y, editor. Tissue engineering for therapeutic use 2. Tokyo: Elsevier; 1998. p. 119–22.
[8] Nakahara T, Nakamura T, Tabata Y, et al. Regeneration of periodontal tissues based on in situ tissue engineering. Inflammation and Regeneration 2003;23(2):116–21 [in Japanese].
[9] Choi SH, Kim CK, Cho KS, et al. Effect of recombinant human bone morphogenetic protein-2/absorbable collagen sponge (rhBMP-2/ACS) on healing in 3-wall intrabony defects in dogs. J Periodontol 2002;73(1):63–72.
[10] Selvig KA, Sorensen RG, Wozney JM, et al. Bone repair following recombinant human bone morphogenetic protein-2 stimulated periodontal regeneration. J Periodontol 2002;73(9): 1020–9.
[11] Huang KK, Shen C, Chiang CY, et al. Effects of bone morphogenetic protein-6 on periodontal wound healing in a fenestration defect of rats. J Periodontal Res 2005;40(1):1–10.
[12] Giannobile WV, Ryan S, Shih MS, et al. Recombinant human osteogenic protein-1 (OP-1) stimulates periodontal wound healing in class III furcation defects. J Periodontol 1998;69(2): 129–37.
[13] Sorensen RG, Polimeni G, Kinoshita A, et al. Effect of recombinant human bone morphogenetic protein-12 (rhBMP-12) on regeneration of periodontal attachment following tooth replantation in dogs. J Clin Periodontol 2004;31(8):654–61.
[14] Tatakis DN, Wikesjo UM, Razi SS, et al. Periodontal repair in dogs: effect of transforming growth factor-beta 1 on alveolar bone and cementum regeneration. J Clin Periodontol 2000; 27(9):698–704.
[15] Murakami S, Takayama S, Kitamura M, et al. Recombinant human basic fibroblast growth factor (bFGF) stimulates periodontal regeneration in class II furcation defects created in beagle dogs. J Periodontal Res 2003;38(1):97–103.
[16] Nevins M, Camelo M, Nevins ML, et al. Periodontal regeneration in humans using recombinant human platelet-derived growth factor-BB (rhPDGF-BB) and allogenic bone. J Periodontol 2003;74(9):1282–92.

[17] Marx RE, Carlson ER, Eichstaedt RM, et al. Platelet-rich plasma: growth factor enhancement for bone grafts. Oral Surg Oral Med Oral Pathol Oral Radiol Endod 1998;85(6): 638–46.

[18] de Obarrio JJ, Arauz-Dutari JI, Chamberlain TM, et al. The use of autologous growth factors in periodontal surgical therapy: platelet gel biotechnology–case reports. Int J Periodontics Restorative Dent 2000;20(5):486–97.

[19] Camargo PM, Lekovic V, Weinlaender M, et al. Platelet-rich plasma and bovine porous bone mineral combined with guided tissue regeneration in the treatment of intrabony defects in humans. J Periodontal Res 2002;37(4):300–6.

[20] Shanaman R, Filstein MR, Danesh-Meyer MJ. Localized ridge augmentation using GBR and platelet-rich plasma: case reports. Int J Periodontics Restorative Dent 2001;21(4):345–55.

[21] Froum SJ, Wallace SS, Tarnow DP, et al. Effect of platelet-rich plasma on bone growth and osseointegration in human maxillary sinus grafts: three bilateral case reports. Int J Periodontics Restorative Dent 2002;22(1):45–53.

[22] Gruber R, Varga F, Fischer MB, et al. Platelets stimulate proliferation of bone cells: involvement of platelet-derived growth factor, microparticles and membranes. Clin Oral Implants Res 2002;13(5):529–35.

[23] Lucarelli E, Beccheroni A, Donati D, et al. Platelet-derived growth factors enhance proliferation of human stromal stem cells. Biomaterials 2003;24(18):3095–100.

[24] Okuda K, Kawase T, Momose M, et al. Platelet-rich plasma contains high levels of platelet-derived growth factor and transforming growth factor-beta and modulates the proliferation of periodontally related cells in vitro. J Periodontol 2003;74(6):849–57.

[25] Frechette JP, Martineau I, Gagnon G. Platelet-rich plasmas: growth factor content and roles in wound healing. J Dent Res 2005;84(5):434–9.

[26] Tabata Y, Ikada Y. Protein release from gelatin matrices. Adv Drug Deliv Rev 1998;31(3): 287–301.

[27] Luginbuehl V, Meinel L, Merkle HP, et al. Localized delivery of growth factors for bone repair. Eur J Pharm Biopharm 2004;58(2):197–208.

[28] Nakahara T, Nakamura T, Kobayashi E, et al. Novel approach to regeneration of periodontal tissues based on in situ tissue engineering: effects of controlled release of basic fibroblast growth factor from a sandwich membrane. Tissue Eng 2003;9(1):153–62.

[29] Nakahara T, Nakamura T, Kobayashi E, et al. Novel approach to regeneration of periodontal tissues based on in situ tissue engineering: effects of controlled release of basic fibroblast growth factor from a sandwich membrane. Clinical Research in Dentistry 2004;1(2):68–77 [in Japanese].

[30] Richardson TP, Peters MC, Ennett AB, et al. Polymeric system for dual growth factor delivery. Nat Biotechnol 2001;19(11):1029–34.

[31] Cao R, Brakenhielm E, Pawliuk R, et al. Angiogenic synergism, vascular stability and improvement of hind-limb ischemia by a combination of PDGF-BB and FGF-2. Nat Med 2003;9(5):604–13.

[32] Pittenger MF, Mackay AM, Beck SC, et al. Multilineage potential of adult human mesenchymal stem cells. Science 1999;284(5411):143–7.

[33] Zuk PA, Zhu M, Mizuno H, et al. Multilineage cells from human adipose tissue: implications for cell-based therapies. Tissue Eng 2001;7(2):211–28.

[34] Korbling M, Estrov Z. Adult stem cells for tissue repair—a new therapeutic concept? N Engl J Med 2003;349(6):570–82.

[35] Petite H, Viateau V, Bensaid W, et al. Tissue-engineered bone regeneration. Nat Biotechnol 2000;18(9):959–63.

[36] Jorgensen C, Gordeladze J, Noel D. Tissue engineering through autologous mesenchymal stem cells. Curr Opin Biotechnol 2004;15(5):406–10.

[37] van Dijk LJ, Schakenraad JM, van der Voort HM, et al. Cell-seeding of periodontal ligament fibroblasts. A novel technique to create new attachment. A pilot study. J Clin Periodontol 1991;18(3):196–9.

[38] Lang H, Schuler N, Nolden R. Attachment formation following replantation of cultured cells into periodontal defects—a study in minipigs. J Dent Res 1998;77(2):393–405.

[39] Dogan A, Ozdemir A, Kubar A, et al. Assessment of periodontal healing by seeding of fibroblast-like cells derived from regenerated periodontal ligament in artificial furcation defects in a dog: a pilot study. Tissue Eng 2002;8(2):273–82.

[40] Nakahara T, Nakamura T, Kobayashi E, et al. In situ tissue engineering of periodontal tissues by seeding with periodontal ligament-derived cells. Tissue Eng 2004;10(3–4): 537–44.

[41] Nakahara T, Nakamura T, Kobayashi E, et al. In situ tissue engineering of periodontal tissues by seeding with periodontal ligament-derived cells. Clinical Research in Dentistry [in Japanese] 2005;2(2):28–34.

[42] Kawaguchi H, Hirachi A, Hasegawa N, et al. Enhancement of periodontal tissue regeneration by transplantation of bone marrow mesenchymal stem cells. J Periodontol 2004;75(9): 1281–7.

[43] Akizuki T, Oda S, Komaki M, et al. Application of periodontal ligament cell sheet for periodontal regeneration: a pilot study in beagle dogs. J Periodontal Res 2005;40(3):245–51.

[44] Yang J, Yamato M, Kohno C, et al. Cell sheet engineering: recreating tissues without biodegradable scaffolds. Biomaterials 2005;26(33):6415–22.

[45] Lekic PC, Rajshankar D, Chen H, et al. Transplantation of labeled periodontal ligament cells promotes regeneration of alveolar bone. Anat Rec 2001;262(2):193–202.

[46] Seo BM, Miura M, Gronthos S, et al. Investigation of multipotent postnatal stem cells from human periodontal ligament. Lancet 2004;364(9429):149–55.

[47] Shea LD, Smiley E, Bonadio J, et al. DNA delivery from polymer matrices for tissue engineering. Nat Biotechnol 1999;17(6):551–4.

[48] Gamradt SC, Lieberman JR. Genetic modification of stem cells to enhance bone repair. Ann Biomed Eng 2004;32(1):136–47.

[49] Gafni Y, Turgeman G, Liebergal M, et al. Stem cells as vehicles for orthopedic gene therapy. Gene Ther 2004;11(4):417–26.

[50] Jin QM, Anusaksathien O, Webb SA, et al. Gene therapy of bone morphogenetic protein for periodontal tissue engineering. J Periodontol 2003;74(2):202–13.

[51] Jin Q, Anusaksathien O, Webb SA, et al. Engineering of tooth-supporting structures by delivery of PDGF gene therapy vectors. Mol Ther 2004;9(4):519–26.

[52] Bonadio J, Smiley E, Patil P, et al. Localized, direct plasmid gene delivery in vivo: prolonged therapy results in reproducible tissue regeneration. Nat Med 1999;5(7):753–9.

[53] Edwards PC, Ruggiero S, Fantasia J, et al. Sonic hedgehog gene-enhanced tissue engineering for bone regeneration. Gene Ther 2005;12(1):75–86.

[54] Ohazama A, Modino SA, Miletich I, et al. Stem-cell-based tissue engineering of murine teeth. J Dent Res 2004;83(7):518–22.

[55] Duailibi MT, Duailibi SE, Young CS, et al. Bioengineered teeth from cultured rat tooth bud cells. J Dent Res 2004;83(7):523–8.

[56] Zhang S. Fabrication of novel biomaterials through molecular self-assembly. Nat Biotechnol 2003;21(10):1171–8.

[57] Bao G, Suresh S. Cell and molecular mechanics of biological materials. Nat Mater 2003; 2(11):715–25.

[58] Li WJ, Tuli R, Huang X, et al. Multilineage differentiation of human mesenchymal stem cells in a three-dimensional nanofibrous scaffold. Biomaterials 2005;26(25):5158–66.

[59] Murphy WL, Simmons CA, Kaigler D, et al. Bone regeneration via a mineral substrate and induced angiogenesis. J Dent Res 2004;83(3):204–10.

[60] Yeong WY, Chua CK, Leong KF, et al. Rapid prototyping in tissue engineering: challenges and potential. Trends Biotechnol 2004;22(12):643–52.

[61] Hutmacher DW, Sittinger M, Risbud MV. Scaffold-based tissue engineering: rationale for computer-aided design and solid free-form fabrication systems. Trends Biotechnol 2004; 22(7):354–62.

[62] Schantz JT, Hutmacher DW, Lam CX, et al. Repair of calvarial defects with customised tissue-engineered bone grafts II. Evaluation of cellular efficiency and efficacy in vivo. Tissue Eng 2003;9(Suppl 1):S127–39.

[63] Warnke PH, Springer IN, Wiltfang J, et al. Growth and transplantation of a custom vascularised bone graft in a man. Lancet 2004;364(9436):766–70.

[64] Gronthos S, Mankani M, Brahim J, et al. Postnatal human dental pulp stem cells (DPSCs) in vitro and in vivo. Proc Natl Acad Sci USA 2000;97(25):13625–30.

[65] Miura M, Gronthos S, Zhao M, et al. SHED: stem cells from human exfoliated deciduous teeth. Proc Natl Acad Sci USA 2003;100(10):5807–12.

[66] Lutolf MP, Hubbell JA. Synthetic biomaterials as instructive extracellular microenvironments for morphogenesis in tissue engineering. Nat Biotechnol 2005;23(1):47–55.

[67] Shi S, Bartold P, Miura M, et al. The efficacy of mesenchymal stem cells to regenerate and repair dental structures. Orthod Craniofac Res 2005;8(3):191–9.

[68] Rahaman MN, Mao JJ. Stem cell-based composite tissue constructs for regenerative medicine. Biotechnol Bioeng 2005;91(3):261–84.

ELSEVIER
SAUNDERS

Dent Clin N Am 50 (2006) 277–298

THE DENTAL
CLINICS
OF NORTH AMERICA

The Impact of Bioactive Molecules to Stimulate Tooth Repair and Regeneration as Part of Restorative Dentistry

Michel Goldberg[a,*], Sally Lacerda-Pinheiro[a,b],
Nadege Jegat[a], Ngampis Six[a],
Dominique Septier[a], Fabienne Priam[a],
Mireille Bonnefoix[a], Kevin Tompkins[c],
Hélène Chardin[a], Pamela Denbesten[d],
Arthur Veis[c], Anne Poliard[b]

[a]*Laboratoire de Réparation et Remodelage des Tissus Oro-Faciaux,
Groupe Matrices Extracellulaires et Biomineralisations, Faculté de Chirurgie Dentaire,
Université René Descartes, Montrouge, France*
[b]*Laboratoire de Differenciation Cellulaire et Prions, Villejuif, France*
[c]*Department of Cell and Molecular Biology, Northwestern University Medical School,
Chicago, IL, USA*
[d]*Growth and Development Department, University of California at San Francisco,
San Francisco, CA, USA*

For years, dental surgeons have used a limited number of capping agents to keep teeth alive. The most efficient was calcium hydroxide. Lessons from developmental biology have provided a better understanding of the genes involved in normal and pathologic processes. Added to an arsenal of transcription factors, growth factors and a series of extracellular matrix (ECM) molecules pave the road for controlled tissue repair and regeneration. These bioactive molecules constitute a large family that will provide

This work was supported by grants from the French Institute of Health and Medical Research/Centre National de la Recherche Scientifique (INSERM/CNRS) (Ingénierie tissulair program) and the French Institut for Dental Research (IFRO).

* Corresponding author. Faculté de Chirurgie Dentaire, Université René Descartes, 1, rue Maurice Arnoux, 92120 Montrouge, France.

E-mail address: mgoldod@aol.com (M. Goldberg).

the tools to modify everyday practice in dentistry substantially in the near future. The investigations discussed in this article are aimed at promoting the healing or regeneration of dental pulp which, in this context, either forms a mineralized barrier of limited size (the so-called "reparative dentinal bridge") or induces a more extensive mineralization area, with the prospect of filling the crown and root pulp partially or totally. The effects of a few ECM molecules have been investigated with these aims. The authors have used them in vivo, in an animal model developed in their laboratory (Fig. 1A), and in vitro, on clonal cell lines of odontoblast precursors obtained from mouse embryo transgenic for an adenovirus-SV40 recombinant plasmid. The effects induced by bioactive molecules on the pulp and on cells are under investigation, and this report summarizes the effects of direct implantation of these cells in the pulp. This review summarizes the experimental approaches performed by the authors' group, with greatly appreciated contributions from a network of collaborators.

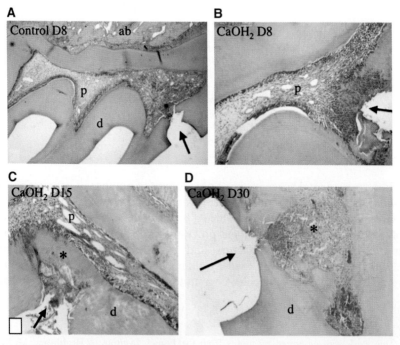

Fig. 1. (A) Eight days after the preparation of the cavity and pulp exposure (D8), an inflammatory process is seen in the mesial part of the pulp chamber. (B) At day 8 (D8), pulp capping with calcium hydroxide induces a limited reaction; (C) 2 weeks (D15) after capping, a reparative dentin bridge starts to be formed (*); and (D) after 1 month (D30), a thick heterogenous dentin bridge fills the mesial part of the pulp (*). The arrow indicates the cavity that has been prepared and location of the pulp exposure. ab, alveolar bone; d, dentin; p, pulp.

A brief historical survey

Calcium hydroxide: cellular mechanisms leading to the formation of a dentinal bridge

For more than 60 years, dental surgeons have used calcium hydroxide as a direct capping agent to induce the formation of a reparative dentinal bridge. In doing so, this bioactive material contributes to the repair of a pulp exposure [1]. Indirect capping with calcium hydroxide used as cavity liner contributes to the formation of reactionary dentin. The reaction is the result of the biologic properties of Ca_2OH_2. As a pulp-capping agent, the high alkaline pH of the preparation induces a burn of limited amplitude at the surface of the pulp exposure. Below the scar, within a few days and when the inflammatory process starts to be resolved, reparative cells are recruited in the central part of the pulp (see Fig. 1B). A first cell division then occurs in the central part of the pulp. The two daughter cells migrate toward the wounded area, where a second cell division occurs [2]. Fully differentiated odontoblasts, which are postmitotic cells, do not participate in these events, and there is evidence that adult resident stem cells that have properties in common with bone-marrow stem cells initiate this process [3–5]. Another possibility is that cell phenotype plasticity allows some cells, already differentiated, to dedifferentiate and then redifferentiate into odontoblast-like or osteoblast-like cells. Therefore, the so-called "pulp stem cells" are more likely multipotent or intermediary undifferentiated cells. This does not exclude the possibility that endothelial cells, pericytes, and pulp fibroblasts also may be candidates for contributing to the population of cells that are recruited, and this constitutes the first step in a series of events that are not understood fully. Cell proliferation is the second event. When a sufficient number of cells is obtained to cover the whole surface that has to be repaired, the cells start their final differentiation.

The reparative process long has been considered as resulting from odontoblast-like cell activity. These cells also are termed neo-odontoblasts or third-generation odontoblasts. There is evidence that at the beginning of the reparative bridge construction, newly differentiated osteoblasts contribute to osteodentin formation (see Fig. 1C, D). At a later stage, and after a terminal phase of polarization, osteoblast/odontoblast precursors become odontoblast-like cells, expressing molecules that are shared by bone and dentin. Actual identification of the terminal phenotype of cells involved in reparative dentin formation is difficult, because the cell types cannot be distinguished easily and they differ only by the level of expression of some ECM molecules. For example, the dentin sialophosphoprotein (DSPP) has been considered a molecule expressed exclusively by odontoblasts and, therefore, a phenotypic marker. Now, DSPP, which is secreted and split immediately into dentin sialoprotein (DSP) and dentin phosphoprotein (DPP), is known to be expressed not exclusively by odontoblasts but also by osteoblasts in a 1:400 ratio [6]. This lack of specific markers renders the precise identification of the reparative cells difficult.

Whatever the biologic agent that stimulates reparative dentin formation, an ECM molecule or a growth factor, and whatever the type of cells implicated in the process, the three successive steps (described previously)—recruitment, proliferation, and differentiation—all are required. Long after the introduction of calcium hydroxide in dental therapies, the effects of other bioactive molecules were investigated. In the early 1990s, Rutherford and coworkers [7,8] demonstrated that indirect capping with bone morphogenetic protein (BMP)-7, also named osteogenic protein (OP-1), was able to stimulate the formation of either reactionary dentin or, as direct capping agent, reparative osteodentin in the root canal of monkeys. These pioneering studies have opened new avenues for regenerative biologic therapies.

A few definitions

To avoid misunderstandings, a consensus has to be reached on definitions. Reactionary dentin results from the stimulation of odontoblasts after carious decay or after the preparation of a cavity. The subodontoblast cell layer, the so-called "Höhl's layer," also may produce a similar beneficial reaction. Beneath a calciotraumatic line, a layer of tubular dentin is formed, more or less in continuity with the dentin formed previously in nonpathologic conditions. Although the staining agent "stains all" that is used to visualize phosphorylated molecules, it interacts only weakly with reactionary dentin, suggesting reduced phosphorylation of the dentin matrix; the structure of this dentin apparently is normal [9].

Reparative dentin formation is under the control of events described previously. Some pulp cells produce it exclusively. If a wound is superficial, such as in a small accidental exposure during the preparation of a cavity, again the subodontoblastic layer, Höhl's layer, may be involved in the repair process. If a dentin carious process has reached the pulp or if the pulp exposure is large, the odontoblasts and the subodontoblastic layer are destroyed. In this case, reparative pulp cells are recruited, proliferate, and, after differentiation, are implicated in the formation of an atubular or osteodentin structure. The terminology used to describe the different types of dentin reflects the similarities between osteodentin and bone where osteocytes are located within lacunae. In contrast, in orthodentin, highly differentiated and polarized odontoblasts display cell bodies that are not embedded in the mineralized tissue but always are located beneath the predentin and at the periphery of the pulp. Protracted odontoblast processes alone are anchored inside the lumen of the tubules in dentin and may extend up to the dentin-enamel junction. The biologic differences between reactionary and reparative dentin are established clearly [10].

New molecules, new approaches, and concepts

The biologic properties, a putative role of BMPs or transforming growth factor-beta (TGF-β), and their putative role in dentin repair led to several studies to determine the effects of these molecules on dentin repair [11–15]. These studies conclude that BMPs or TGF-β may induce reparative dentin formation. Gene expression was found in human and animal dental pulps for BMPs and for their receptors [16–19]. They both probably contribute to the beneficial reaction. The intimate mechanisms mediating this action remain obscure, however.

Two major views arise from the available literature. First, there is converging evidence that reparative processes recapitulate early developmental events that lead to dental tissue formation [20]. In support of this mechanism, c-jun and jun-B proto-oncogenes [21] and the Delta-Notch signaling normally expressed at early stages of tooth development [22] are re-expressed during pulp healing. This suggests that transcription factors, growth factors, or ECM molecules may contribute to promote reparative dentin formation or, moreover, promote partial or total pulp mineralization. Pioneering investigations already are undertaken that support this mechanism [23–25].

Second, it seems important to mention a few points regarding the potential multifunctional nature of ECM molecules. This multifunctionality is a well-accepted concept that has to be taken into account in the interpretation of many studies. For a long time, the paradigm was that one molecule plays one single role. According to this way of thinking, a molecule recognized as a member of the ECM is involved in the tissue structure alone. The concept recently has been revisited or modified, and it is now well recognized that most molecules display more than one function.

For example, native collagen subunit association is regulated by the cleavage of the C-terminal nonhelicoidal extensions by a C-procollagen peptidase involved in the processing of a structural protein. The C-proteinase also was identified as a BMP-1, a molecule that is a growth factor [26]. In this specific case, the enzyme has two different functions.

As another example of multifunctionality, for years amelogenin was considered a molecule implicated only in enamel formation. Most studies were devoted to the structural aspect of the molecule. With the discovery of the spliced forms of small molecular weight amelogenins arose the perception that such amelogenin gene splice products have potential signaling properties [27]. Enamelysin (matrix metalloproteinase-20 [MMP-20]) also is expressed in cells that are not ameloblasts and, therefore, not implicated in enamel formation. These two examples suggest either that isoforms of a family of molecules obtained by alternative splicing may play different biologic roles or that after partial degradation, residual peptides may be converted in an activated form and display functional properties hidden in the intact molecule. This sheds light on the complex effects of ECM implanted in a given tissue to promote healing or regeneration.

Consequently, molecules involved in embryonic development may be used as reparative or regenerating agents. This is a result not only of the intrinsic properties of the molecules to rejuvenate a tissue but also of the multifunctionality of such bioactive molecules.

In the course of these investigations, two different approaches have been used. Various ECM molecules were implanted in exposed pulp tissue, anticipating that some cells would be specifically recruited, would proliferate, and finally would differentiate into cells involved in the formation of reparative dentin. Preliminary results have been obtained with a second approach involving clonal pulp cells that produce, after direct implantation in a target zone, a specific ECM capable in some cases of mineralizing further.

Dentin matrix proteins composition, functions, and bioactive potentials

Dentin is a complex tissue, produced mostly by odontoblasts. Many ECM molecules already are identified. Some are associated with the mineralization process or initiation of the crystal formation or crystal growth, whereas others are acting as inhibitors (Table 1).

Recent studies demonstrate the complex biologic effects of some ECM components. They are mineralization promoters or inhibitors, but they also play a role in cell differentiation. For example, such dual functions are reported for DPP, also named phosphophoryn, a molecule that triggers dentin mineralization and regulates the gene expression and differentiation of a mouse osteoblastic cell line, a mouse fibroblastic cell line, and human mesenchymal stem cells via the integrin/mitogen-activated protein kinase (MAPK) signaling pathway [28]. Therefore, in addition to the well-documented role in mineral nucleation, DPP plays a role in cell differentiation and other novel signaling functions. Along the same lines, overexpression of dentin matrix protein (DMP)-1 induces the differentiation of embryonic mesenchymal cells to odontoblast-like cells [29]. DMP-1 is regulated by c-fos and c-jun transcription factors and plays a role in early osteoblast differentiation [30]. Signaling effects also are well documented with the amelogenin gene splice products, A+4 and A−4 [27]. The complexity is enhanced by the fact that matrix molecules are substrates for MMPs or for metalloproteinases, and fragments of the processed proteins may be biologically active. For example, DMP-1 is processed physiologically by BMP-1/tolloid-like proteinases [31]. DSP and amelogenin are substrates for MMP-2 [32]. Dentin mineralization and enamel formation are impaired by inhibitors of MMPs [32,33]

Although the concept of a pulp-dentin complex has been developed, the composition of the dental pulp differs from dentin. Table 2 summarizes the pulp ECM composition, which differs substantially from that of dentin. In addition, most of the molecules associated with the mineralization process are absent or present in minute amounts. Therefore, implantation of such molecules into the dental pulp involves introducing an exogenous protein.

Table 1
Composition and properties of the extracellular matrix molecules located in dentin and, therefore, involved in dentinogenesis

Molecules synthesized by odontoblasts

Collagens, 90% type I (90%), including type I trimer (11%), type III (1%–3%), type V (1%–3%)	Constitute a scaffold (may be used as a scaffold or a carrier for bioactive molecules)	3-D–network indirectly implicated in dentin or pulp mineralization
Noncollagenous proteins, 10% Phosphorylated molecules SIBLINGs		
	DSPP 72-kd mice, 90–95-kd rat, 155-kd bovine, cleaved into DSP (N-terminal) (53 kd) and DPP (C-terminal):large amount of aspatic acid, phosphoserine, initiator and modulator of dentin apatite crystal formation	Chromosome 4, locus q20–21, *Dspp* gene defect is associated with dentinogenesis imperfecta DSP: 6 Pi/mol DPP: ~209 Pi/mol
	DMP-1 (61 kd), activation of OC	Chromosome 4, q20–21 473 aa, proteolytically processed into 37-kd (N-terminal) and 57-kd (C-terminal) fragments
	#Bone acidic glycoprotein (BAG75), 75 kd	
	BSP (75 kd) Nucleator of initial apatite crystals, inhibitor of the growth of crystals, attachment molecule (RGD), collagen fibrillation	Chromosome 4, q20–21 303 aa, 5.85 Pi/mol
	OPN (44 kd), RGD sequence, polyaspatic acid motifs Inhibitor of HaP formation	Chromosome 4, q20–21 301 aa, 13 Pi/mol Chromosome 4, locus 4q21
	MEPE	Mineralization inhibitor
	56.6 kd = osteocyte factor (OF45)	A peptide fragment containing the RGD and SGDG sequence stimulate bone formation

(continued on next page)

Table 1 (*continued*)

Molecules synthesized by odontoblasts		
Other phosphorylated matrix proteins	Amelogenins (spliced forms) A−4 (6.9 kd) and A+4 (8.1 kd), phosphorylated in Ser16 of the RAP domain (N-terminal)	Chromosomes x and y Signaling molecules
	Small leucine-rich proteoglycans (SLRP) CS/DS Decorin = biglycan: 40 kd	Decorin and biglycan may be phosphorylated Contribute to dentin mineralization
Nonphosphorylated proteins	KS SLRP: fibromodulin (42 kd), lumican (38 kd), osteoadherin (42 kd)	Repressor mineralization?
	OC (5.7–6.8 kd), a member of the γ-carboxyglutamic acid containing (gla-) protein family (10–12.7 kd)	Expressed by odontoblasts: adhesion, mineralization inhibitor?
	Osteonectin (= SPARC protein = BM40) (43 kd)	Mineralization inhibitor?
Enzymes		
Metalloproteinases	MMPs: MMP-1, MMP-2, MMP-9, MMP-3, MMP-20 MT1-MMP TIMPs 1–3	Collagenase, gelatinases, stromelysin 1, enamelysin
Others enzymes	Serine proteases, acid phosphatase, alkaline phosphatase	
Growth factors	TGF-β1, insulin-like growth factors I and II	
Proteins taking origin from the serum, not synthesized by odontoblasts	α2HS glycoprotein (50 kd) Albumin	Present exclusively in mineralized tissues Lipid carrier
Lipids		
Membrane lipids	66%	Related to dentin mineralization (crystal ghosts)
Lipids associated with the mineralized phase	33% acidic phospholipids	

Abbreviations: #, very similar to; CS/DS, chondroitin sulfate/dermatan sulfate; HS, heparan sulfate; KS, keratan sulfate; TGF-β1, transforming growth factor-beta 1; TIMP, tissue inhibitor of metalloproteinase.

Table 2
Extracellular matrix components of the dental pulp

Collagens, 34% of the whole	Type I, 56%	
	Type III, 41%	
	Type V, 1%–3%	
	Type IV	
	Type VI and fibrillin	
Noncollagenous proteins	Large proteoglycans	CS/DS, KS, HS: versican
	Small leucine-rich	Decorin, biglycan
	proteoglycans	Two forms: cellular and
	Fibronectin	fibronectin taking origin
	Elastin	from the blood serum
	MMPs	MMP-1, MMP-2, MMP-9,
		MMP-3, MMP-20
Inflammatory molecules	Interleukin-1,	
	prostaglandins,	
	vasoactive intestinal	
	polypeptide-like	
Growth factors	TGF-β1, BMP-2,	
	BMP-4, BMP-6	
Growth factor receptors	BMPR-I	Activin receptor-like kinase-1
		(ALK-1), ALK-2, BMPR-1A,
		ALK-4, ALK-5, ALK-6,
		or BMP 1B
	BMPR-II	Type II receptor of BMP
Cellular and extracellular		Phospholipids
matrix lipids		
Molecules that are	No OC, no osteonectine,	
not present	no DPP, no DSP,	
or are present	no DMP-1, no BSP	
in minute amounts	(traces of sialoprotein)	

The properties of a few of these molecules suggest their potential as inducers of mineralized tissues, taking into account the known composition of the dental tissues and the data available on in vivo distribution and in vitro effects in cell free systems or in cell cultures. To this end, the authors established a reliable animal model to study the stimulation of pulp repair, then explored the effects of implantation of bone sialoprotein (BSP), OP-1, Dentonin (a peptide of matrix extracellular phosphoglycoprotein [MEPE]), and two spliced forms of dentin amelogenins (A+4 and A−4) in the exposed pulp of rat molar. In a second strategy, the authors performed in vitro studies on odontoblast progenitor cell lines corresponding to different steps of differentiation. This strategy allowed characterizing by reverse transcription–polymerase chain reaction (RT-PCR) the short-term effects of bioactive molecules on the level of expression of some genes and transcription factors—such as Runx2, Pax9, Msx1, and Msx2—and ECM molecules—such as type II collagen, osteocalcin (OC), and DSP. These odontoblast precursors also were implanted in the pulp.

Mechanisms involved in the in vivo reparative processes

The in vivo model of exposed rat molar pulp

In 1990, Ohshima [34] described the changes in odontoblasts and pulp capillaries after cavity preparation in the rat maxillary molar. The cavity was prepared in the mesial aspect of the first maxillary molar. The authors modified this experimental protocol by using electrosurgery to remove the gingival papilla before any cavity preparation. This allows a more consistent preparation of half moon cavities in the cervical area of the rat molar. This location avoids interference with the pulp horns, which biologically are different in the enamel free area from the rest of the pulp chamber. Secondly, this cervical location allows a better mechanical resistance to occlusal pressures and, consequently, fewer restorative fillings with glass ionomer cements (GIC) are lost. The cavity is drilled with carbide burs in fewer than 2 seconds. The preparation of the cavity and its filling with a GIC induce only a slight inflammatory reaction [35]. The residual dentin then is pushed with a steel probe, which allows obtaining a pulp exposure of limited size. This process avoids stretching of the pulp tissue around the bur and uncontrolled pulp damages. The projection of dentin debris inside the pulp may release ECM molecules, however, contributing to spontaneous pulp healing with the resultant formation of reparative dentin [23–25]. In spite of this complication, this system provides an excellent animal model for study of the effects of bioactive molecules on the dental pulp [36].

Experimental results: in vivo and in vitro approaches

Bone sialoprotein/collagen implantation

Among the dentin ECM that seems to display intrinsic bioactive properties for promoting the formation of a reparative tissue, BSP is a good candidate. Implantation of the molecule in calvaria leads to rapid repair of a critical defect greater than or equal to 8 mm, with stimulation of the recruitment of bone forming cells, which differentiate and subsequently form a small amount of cartilage, replaced by bone [37–39]. In addition, BSP is a phosphorylated protein with tyrosine sulphatation and an arginine-glycine-aspartate (RGD) attachment sequence. Several stretches of polyglutamic acid are involved in binding to hydroxyapatite [40]. BSP enhances the fibrillogenesis of collagen [41]. BSP messenger RNA is expressed by odontoblasts of the incisor during dentinogenesis, and a polyclonal antibody directed against BSP reacts positively with epitopes located in odontoblast cell bodies and processes and with the peritubular dentin [42,43]. In addition, pulp cells do not express BSP.

Eight days after the implantation of BSP with gelatin as a carrier, an inflammatory process was seen (Fig. 2A). Some loci of mineralization appeared around the dentin fragments that were pushed into the pulp

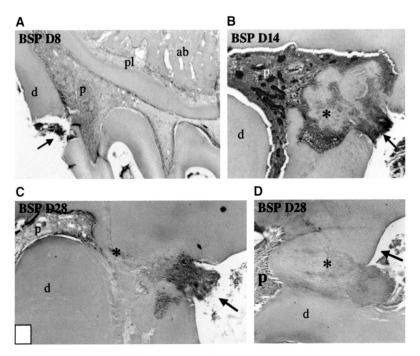

Fig. 2. (A) Implantation of BSP leads to an initial moderate inflammatory pulp reaction after 8 days (D8); (B) the reaction is not resolved after 2 weeks (D14). The formation of reparative dentin starts around dentin debris that has been pushed into the pulp during pulp exposure. (C, D) After 1 month (D28), a dense and homogeneous reparative dentin formation (*) fills the mesial part of the pulp totally. The arrow indicates the cavity that has been prepared and location of the pulp exposure. ab, alveolar bone; d, dentin; p, pulp; pl, periodontal ligament.

during the preparation of the teeth at 14 days (see Fig. 2B). After 1 month, the mesial part of the pulp chamber was filled with a homogeneous atubular dentin (see Fig. 2C, D). Inflammatory processes were resolved [36]. In the controls, after calcium hydroxide pulp capping, poorly filled interruptions, appearing as channels, porosities, or large osteodentin areas, were seen, which induce discontinuities in the dentinal bridge. Therefore, protection against possible bacterial recontamination was questionable. The major defect of calcium hydroxide is that long-term evaluations are unable to protect the pulps efficiently. This should not be the case after BSP implantation, because the reparative material is more homogeneous and should lead to a more efficient protection of the pulp.

Bone morphogenetic protein-7 (osteogenic protein-1)/ collagen implantation

BMP-7 (OP-1) is used as a lining agent indirectly promoting the formation of reactionary dentin and is implanted directly in exposed pulp to induce reparative dentin by many groups [7,8,11,12,19,44]. The authors determined the effects of OP-1 in their first rat maxillary molar model for dentin repair [15]. After implantation of OP-1 (1, 3, or 10 μg of recombinant BMP-7/implant) mixed with small collagen pellets, an inflammatory process was observed that was not totally resolved after 1 month. After 30 days, the mesial portion of the coronal pulp was filled with a heterogeneous osteodentin porous material. Globular structures did not merge and interglobular spaces were filled with pulp remnants. Reparative dentin formation was defective in the crown of the teeth (Fig. 3A, B). In contrast, the mesial roots were filled with a homogeneous dense material located beneath a calciotraumatic line. No appearance of lumen of root canal was detectable on serially cut sections.

The striking difference between the coronal and radicular pulp in rats treated with OP-1 was an unexpected result. The differences between the crown and root dentin are documented and understood poorly. During crown formation, the enamel organ that expresses large amounts of amelogenin surrounds the embryonic pulp. The formation of the root is driven by Hertwig's sheath, which does not express amelogenin, although most of other enamel proteins are expressed. In some species, dentin is lacking phosphorylated proteins. Differences also appear with respect to the vascular network and nerve development.

In the crown, radioautographic investigation [2] and proliferation cell nuclear antigen (PCNA) immunodetection provide evidence that reparative cells are recruited in the central part of the coronal pulp and later move toward the lateral area where the reparative process takes place. In the root, an initial localization in the central part is not apparent, but PCNA-labeled cells are seen already in the lateral subodontoblastic area. This provides some explanation of the fact that reparative dentin is deposited along the root canal walls, with a gradual reduction in diameter of the root pulp, leading to complete obliteration of the lumen.

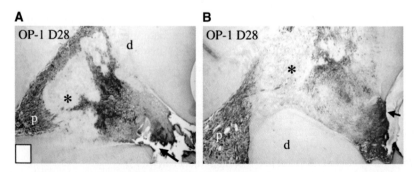

Fig. 3. (*A, B*) One month (D28) after implantation of OP-1, a heterogeneous formation of the osteodentin type fills the mesial part of the pulp chamber (*). Pulp remnants contribute to the heterogeneity of the reparative structure. The arrow indicates the cavity that has been prepared and location of the pulp exposure. d, dentin; p, pulp; pl, periodontal ligament.

Dentonin: a peptide derived of the matrix extracellular phosphorylated glycoprotein

MEPE is a member of the SIBLING (small integrin-binding ligand, N-linked glycoprotein) family [45]. Similar to DMP-1, MEPE has high serine content and contains a hydrophobic leader sequence and RGD and SGDG motifs. It is described as a mineralization inhibitor [46–48]. Dentonin (Acologix, Emeryville, California) (also known as AC-100) is a 23-amino-acid fragment of MEPE that stimulates the proliferation of dental pulp stem cells and their differentiation in vitro [49].

In experiments to determine the effect of MEPE on pulp repair, the authors used another carrier more appropriate for experiments using molecules that are soluble in aqueous culture media, the Affigel (Biorad, Hercules, California) agarose beads (75–150 μm in diameter).

Agarose is a sulphated galactan, which may induce a biologic effect per se. Therefore, a control group was included with the exposed pulp implanted with agarose beads alone. After agarose bead implantation, an inflammatory reaction could be seen at 8 days, but it resolved at 90 days. Some reparative dentin was formed after 15 days. Beneath a reparative dentinal bridge, however, after 90 days coronal pulp still was present and the lumen of the root canal was reduced but pulp tissue remained. Hence, the contribution of agarose beads was not negligible but was restricted compared with the major effects of the bioactive molecules.

The initial recruitment of reparative pulp cells by Dentonin peptides is faster than that with the two previous molecules described previously. At day 8 after implantation, a ring of differentiating cells was located at the periphery of beads. Around the dentin debris pushed during the pulp exposure, precocious mineralization was detectable (Fig. 4A). After 2 weeks, loci of initial mineralization, confluence of mineralization nodules (calcospherites), and massive formation of reparative dentin were observed. The transformation of the mesial coronal pulp into a homogeneous mineralized tissue was slower thereafter. Dentin debris, remnants of the agarose beads, and other materials were embedded into a thick area of reparative dentin occluding largely the coronal pulp (see Fig. 4B). Such events are not detected in the root. Hence, Dentonin seems to be a good inducer of pulp mineralization in vivo.

In vivo implantation of AM+4 and A−4 in the exposed pulp and in an ectopic nonmineralizing gingival tissue: in vitro effects of the amelogenin gene splice products on odontoblast and osteoblast precursors

Implantation in the exposed pulp

A small molecular weight molecule that appeared initially as a chondrogenic-inducing agent was isolated from calf and rat dentin [50]. This molecule was an amelogenin [51]. Soon after, the existence of two small molecular weight amelogenin splice products (A+4 and A−4) was identified

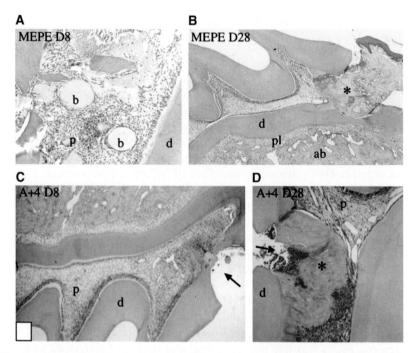

Fig. 4. (*A*) Eight days after implantation of agarose beads (b) loaded with a small fragment of MEPE, an inflammatory process is seen. Cells are grouped around the beads. (*B*) One month after MEPE implantation (D28), a thick reparative dentinal bridge is formed, occluding the pulp exposure. Agarose beads and dentin debris are embedded in the reparative dentin (*). (*C*) Day 8 after implantation in the pulp of agarose beads loaded with A+4. (*D*) One month after A+4 implantation (D28), a thick homogeneous reparative dentinal bridge occludes the pulp exposure. An inflammatory process is not yet resolved in the root canal pulp. The arrow indicates the cavity that has been prepared and location of the pulp exposure. ab, alveolar bone; d, dentin; p, pulp; pl, periodontal ligament.

in an odontoblast library. A+4 is derived from all exons from 1 to 7, but lacks the 5′ sequence of exon 6 to synthesize an 8.1-kd alternatively spliced amelogenin. A−4 was similar to A+4 but did not include exon 4 to produce a 6.9-kd alternatively spliced amelogenin [52]. A+4 induced the rapid expression of the transcription factor Sox9, whereas A−4 elevated the transcription of Cbfa1 [52]. These two spliced forms soaked on agarose beads were implanted in the exposed pulp.

Implantation of A+4 leads to the formation of a thick and homogeneous dentinal bridge. The pulp in the root canal was reduced in diameter as a result of the gradual obstruction of the lumen by reparative dentin. The initial inflammatory process (see Fig. 4C) was decreasing at 15 days, but residual inflammatory process was present 30 days after implantation (see Fig. 4D). No inflammation was detectable after 90 days. At that time, observed beneath a thick dentinal bridge was a pulp reduced in size in the crown and root of the teeth. In some cases, there was no pulp tissue remaining in the mesial root.

Eight days after the implantation of agarose beads loaded with A−4, inflammation was moderate in contrast with the control and the other experimental groups (Fig. 5A). A dense ring of cells was seen around the beads (see Fig. 5B). At day 14, reparative dentin formation was seen in the crown where diffuse mineralization of the pulp was developing rapidly but did not fill the mesial part of the pulp chamber totally (see Fig. 5C). This pulp area was occluded at day 30 with a diffuse mineralized tissue, as shown by studies performed on undemineralized section of molars examined with an electron microprobe combined with a scanning electron microscope. In parallel, at day 14, the lumen of the root canal displayed a reduced diameter as a result of the extensive formation of a homogeneous reparative dentin layer. At day 30, the root canal lumen was not visible and was occluded totally by

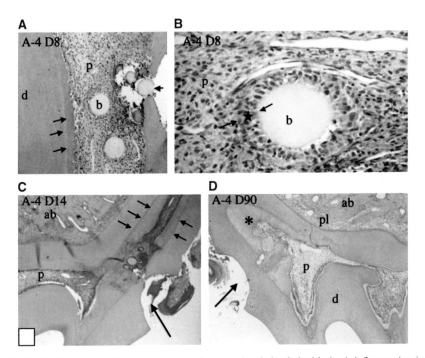

Fig. 5. (*A*) Eight days after implantation of agarose beads loaded with A−4, inflammation is moderate. (*B*) Densely packed around an agarose bead used as A−4 carrier, a ring of cells that underwent terminal differentiation is seen at day 8. (*C*) After 14 days (D14), reparative dentin is forming actively in the mesial part of the pulp. The diameter of the root canal is reduced by the formation of dentin limited by the calciotraumatic lines (*arrows*). (*D*) After 3 months (D90), the mesial pulp chamber and the mesial root canal are totally filled by reparative dentin. The periodontal ligament is maintained in shape and width. Alveolar bone apparently is unchanged. The arrow indicates the cavity that has been prepared and location of the pulp exposure. ab, alveolar bone; d, dentin; p, pulp; pl, periodontal ligament.

a homogeneous mineralized tissue. At day 90, it was seen that the effect of the molecule was limited to the pulp without any alteration of the periodontal ligament (see Fig. 5D).

Using PCNA immunostaining, it was observed that cell proliferation occurred in the central part of the crown pulp, some distance away from the beads (Fig. 6A). In the root, proliferation occurred only in the subodontoblastic area and never in the central part. The ring of cells located around the beads was immunolabeled positively for osteopontin (OPN) and BSP but negatively for DSP (see Fig. 6B, C). This suggests that they are cells differentiating into osteoblast lineage cells. A few cells in the central pulp and beneath the exposure area were found positive for DSP, whereas those located around the beads never displayed any significant labeling (see Fig. 6C). DSP mostly is a dentin protein although expressed at very low level in bone.

After either A+4 or A−4 implantation, two groups of cells differentiated simultaneously, providing odontoblasts near the pulp exposure and osteoblasts in an area located more centrally, which may be implicated in osteodentin formation. Alternatively, it is possible that a single group of cells of the osteoblastic and odontoblastic lineage is recruited and proliferates. Initially located in the central part of the pulp, around the beads, they may migrate from the central part of the pulp toward the peripheral wounded area

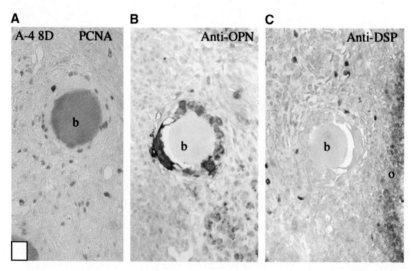

Fig. 6. Eight days (D8) after A−4 implantation in an exposed pulp, cell proliferation is visualized by PCNA staining (*A*). The dividing cells are located some distance away from the bead (*B*). Anti-OPN staining reveals that the cells located around the beads are positively labeled (b), whereas a few cells distributed throughout the central part of the pulp are positively stained with anti-DSP (*C*). They are located some distance away from the bead. DSP antibody stains positively odontoblasts cell bodies (o). The arrow indicates the cavity that has been prepared and location of the pulp exposure.

where they are implicated in reparative dentin formation [2]. Doing so, they apparently shift from an osteoblast phenotype to an odontoblast phenotype. To get a better understanding of the process, the authors investigated the reaction at early time points after implantation (1 and 3 days) [53]. Immunohistochemical data show that cells proliferate (PCNA) at both time points. RP59 is a marker of osteoblast recruitment also detected in primitive mesenchymal cells, erythroid cells, and megacaryocytes. A few pulp cells are RP59 positive at day 3, mostly after stimulation with A−4. The reaction is weaker but still positive with A+4 (Table 3) [54,55].

In vitro effects of A+4 and A−4 on odontoblast progenitors

Because the early events leading to the reparative process are understood poorly, the authors are using RT-PCR to investigate the nature of stimulation with A+4 and A−4 on two clones of odontoblast precursors (described previously) [56]. The two cell lines used reacted to A+4 or A−4, and Sox9 expression was stimulated. Lhx6, a member of the LIM-homeobox–containing genes encoding transcriptional regulators, was expressed transiently at 24 hours, whereas Lhx7 was expressed constantly at 6 hours, 24 hours, and 48 hours but by one clone alone. OC and DSP also were expressed at 48 hours by another odontoblastic clone.

Early effects (6–24 h) were detected on the expression of diverse transcription factors involved in bone cartilage and odontoblast differentiation; then, expression of ECM molecules, such as OC and DSP, was activated (48 h). Differences were noted between the type of cells in their stage of differentiation between the respective effects of A+4 and A−4 and in relation with the time course [57]. This cascade of events suggests the presence of receptors, specific or not, and intracellular signaling pathways now in focus.

In vivo implantation in ectopic site

Because an inflammatory reaction was seen in most of the pulp implantations, the authors wondered whether or not some inflammatory cells could contribute to the process of dentin formation. It is reported that some stem cells take origin from bone marrow [58], whereas others may derive from

Table 3
Immunohistochemical staining found at day 1 (D1) and day 3 (D3) after bead implantation with a marker of proliferation (PCNA), of the osteoblastic recruitment (RP59), OPN, and DSP

	Beads D1	Beads D3	A+4 D1	A+4 D3	A−4 D1	A−4 D3
PCNA	+	−	±	++	±	+++
RP59	+	−	+	±	−	++
OPN	±	+	−	+	±	++
DSP	−	−	−	−	−	−

Note that at the time, DSP is not present, suggesting that cells bearing an odontoblast phenotype are not yet differentiated.

circulating $CD14^+$ monocytes, which may differentiate into osteoblast or chondroblast progenitors [59]. To elucidate if the cells were resident cells or circulating cells, the authors decided to implant agarose beads loaded with A+4 or A−4 in the gingiva of mice, a nonmineralizing tissue where osteoblast and odontoblast progenitors is not expected.

Three days after implantation, a strong inflammatory process was observed in the lamina propria. The inflammatory cells seemed of the leukocyte lineage, as suggested by their $CD45^+$ and $I-A^k$ staining. This inflammatory process was decreased at day 8 and barely detectable at day 30. When beads were loaded with A+4 or A−4, some cells were RP59 positive. These cells also expressed Sox9. PCNA staining was negative, suggesting that the RP59 positive cells are not derived from the proliferation of resident stem cells, rather from the migration of circulating cells with progenitor properties. These cells displayed a positive labeling for BSP and OPN but remained negative for DSP. Despite the fact that these cells expressed molecules considered specific markers of a bone-like mineralized tissue, no mineralization was detected, in contrast with the observations after implantation of the amelogenin peptides in the pulp. This suggests that (1) differentiation of osteogenic precursors is not necessarily dependant on local resident stem cells; (2) the presence of precursors results either from the migration of cells from the bone marrow or circulating monocytes mixed within the inflammatory cell population; (3) the last events leading to a mineralization phenomenon are more specific and seem to be under the control of the tissue; and (4) as reported elsewhere, in in vitro and in vivo [27,52], the two amelogenin peptides, A+4 and A−4, implanted in the dental pulp, have a differential effect.

This set of experiments shows that the amelogenin peptides provide a useful tool for investigating the mechanisms involved in reparative dentin formation and in pulp reaction. Further studies are needed to determine which part of the molecule is active biologically and how this action is mediated.

Prospective area of research: cell recruitment by extracellular matrix or mineralized extracellular matrix produced by osteoblast and odontoblast precursors

Two different strategies have been used. One implants bioactive molecules, and we may expect an appropriate group of cells to be recruited and to proliferate and differentiate into cells that produce an ECM with mineralizing potential. The other one implants odontoblast/osteoblast precursors that promote pulp mineralization. The injection of some of the clones of immortalized odontoblast precursors in the pulp provides interesting preliminary results. The injection of a population of cloned cells [56] in the mouse mandibular incisor induces the formation of a huge area of osteodentin within 11 days (Fig. 7). Further experiments using these cells are currently in progress.

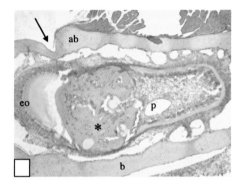

Fig. 7. Eleven days after the injection of odontoblast progenitors cells in the pulp of mouse incisor, together with agarose beads used in this case only to visualize the injection site, reparative dentin is formed massively (*) in the upper part of the pulp, beneath the enamel organ. The arrow indicates the site where the injection of cells and beads was made. The arrow indicates the cavity that has been prepared and location of the pulp exposure. ab, alveolar bone; eo, enamel organ; p, pulp.

In conclusion, the authors have investigated the possible contribution of a series of ECM molecules to the formation of reparative dentin and conclude that BSP (a fragment of MEPE) and some amelogenin gene splice products (A+4 and A−4) stimulate either the formation of a reparative dentinal bridge, the closure of the mesial coronal pulp chamber, or the total closure of the root canal. This choice of bioactive molecules is not exhaustive and others may be used in this context, such as DSP, DPP, or DMP-1. Combined in vivo and in vitro approaches to study the function of amelogenin may contribute to clarifying the biologic cascade of events. Shortcuts may be found by direct implantation of specific cells in the pulp, as this approach also works. These two tissue-engineering strategies may contribute to substantial changes in the concept of promoting healing and regeneration of altered dental tissues.

References

[1] Zander HA. Reaction of the pulp to calcium hydroxide. J Dent Res 1939;18:373–9.
[2] Fitzgerald M, Chiego DJ, Heys DR. Autoradiographic analysis of odontoblast replacement following pulp exposure in primate teeth. Arch Oral Biol 1990;35:707–15.
[3] Gronthos S, Brahim J, Li W, et al. Stem cell properties of human dental pulp stem cells. J Dent Res 2002;81:531–5.
[4] Gronthos S, Mankani M, Brahim J, et al. Postnatal human dental pulp stem cells (DPSCs) in vitro and in vivo. Proc Natl Acad Sci U S A 2000;97:13625–30.
[5] Procop DJ. Marrow stromal cells as stem cells for non hematopoietic tissues. Science 1997; 276:71–4.
[6] Qin C, Brunn JC, Cadena E, et al. Expression of dentin sialophosphoprotein gene in bone. J Dent Res 2002;81:392–4.
[7] Rutherford RB, Wahle J, Tucker M, et al. Induction of reparative dentine formation in monkey by recombinant human osteogenic protein-1. Arch Oral Biol 1993;38:571–6.

[8] Rutherford RB, Spängberg L, Tucker M, et al. The time-course of the induction of repara-tive dentine formation in monkeys by recombinant human osteogenic protein-1. Arch Oral Biol 1994;39:833–8.

[9] Takagi Y, Sasaki S. Histological distribution of phosphophoryn in normal and pathological human dentins. J Oral Pathol 1986;15:463–7.

[10] Lesot H, Bègue-Kirn C, Kübler MD, et al. Experimental induction of odontoblast differentiation and stimulation during reparative processes. Cell Materials 1993;3: 201–17.

[11] Nakashima M. The induction of reparative dentine in the amputated dental pulp of the dog by bone morphogenetic protein. Arch Oral Biol 1990;35:493–7.

[12] Nakashima M. Induction of dentine in amputated pulp of dogs by recombinant human bone morphogenetic proteins-2 and -4 with collagen matrix. Arch Oral Biol 1994;39:1085–9.

[13] Lianjia Y, Yuhao G, White FH. Bovine bone morphogenetic protein-induced dentinogene-sis. Clin Orthop Rel Res 1993;259:305–12.

[14] Tziafas D, Alvanou A, Papadimitriou S, et al. Effects of recombinant basic fibroblast growth factor, insulin-like growth factor-II and transforming growth factor-β1 on dog dental pulp cells in vivo. Arch Oral Biol 1998;43:431–44.

[15] Six N, Lasfargues J-J, Goldberg M. Recombinant human Bone Morphogenetic Protein-7 (Osteogenic Protein-1) induces differential repair responses in the coronal and radicular areas of the exposed rat molar pulp. Arch Oral Biol 2002;47:177–87.

[16] Takeda K, Oida S, Goseki M, et al. Expression of bone morphogenetic protein genes in the human dental pulp cells. Bone 1994;5:467–70.

[17] Takeda K, Oida S, Ichijo H, et al. Molecular cloning of rat morphogenetic protein (BMP) Type IA receptor and its expression during ectopic bone formation induced by BMP. Bio-chem Biophys Res Commun 1994;204:203–9.

[18] Toyono T, Nakashima M, Kuhara S, et al. Expression of TGF-β superfamily receptors in dental pulp. J Dent Res 1997;76:1555–60.

[19] Gu K, Smoke RH, Rutherford RB. Expression of genes for bone morphogenetic proteins and receptors in human dental pulp. Arch Oral Biol 1996;41:919–23.

[20] Mitsiadis TA, Rahiotis C. Parallels between tooth development and repair: conserved molecular mechanisms following carious and dental injury. J Dent Res 2004;83: 896–902.

[21] Kitamura C, Kimura K, Nakayama T, et al. Temporal and spatial expression of c-jun and jun-B proto-oncogenes in pulp cells involved with reparative dentinogenesis after cavity preparation of rat molars. J Dent Res 1999;78:673–80.

[22] Mitsiadis TA, Fried K, Goridis C. Reactivation of Delta-Notch signaling after injury: com-plementary expression patterns of ligant and receptor in dental pulp. Exp Cell Res 1999;246: 312–8.

[23] Tziafas D, Kolokuris I, Alvanou A, et al. Short term dentinogenic response of dog dental pulp tissue after its induction by demineralized or native dentine or predentine. Arch Oral Biol 1992;37:119–28.

[24] Smith AJ, Tobias RS, Cassidy N, et al. Odontoblast stimulation in ferrets by dentin matrix components. Arch Oral Biol 1994;39:13–22.

[25] Takata T, D'Errico JA, Atkins KB, et al. Protein extracts of dentin affect proliferation and differentiation of osteoprogenitor cells in vitro. J Periodontol 1998;69:1247–55.

[26] Li S-W, Sieron AL, Fertala A, et al. The C-proteinase that processes procollagens to fibrillar collagens is identical to the protein previously identified as bone morphogenetic protein-1. Proc Natl Acad Sci U S A 1996;93:5127–30.

[27] Veis A. Amelogenin gene splice products: potential signaling molecules. Cell Mol Life Sci 2003;60:38–55.

[28] Jadlowiec J, Koch H, Zhang X, et al. Phosphoryn regulates the gene expression and differ-entiation of NIH3T3, MC3T3-E1, and human mesenchymal stem cells via the integrin/ MAPK signaling pathway. J Biol Chem 2004;279:53323–30.

[29] Narayanan K, Srinivas R, Ramachandran A, et al. Differentiation of embryonic mesenchymal cells to odontoblast-like cells by overexpression of dentin matrix protein 1. Proc Natl Acad Sci U S A 2001;98:4516–21.

[30] Narayanan K, Srinivas R, Peterson MC, et al. Transcriptional regulation of dentin matrix protein 1 by JunB and p300 during osteoblast differentiation. J Biol Chem 2004;279: 44294–302.

[31] Steiglitz BM, Ayala M, Narayanan K, et al. Bone morphogenetic protein-1/Tolloid-like proteinases process dentin matrix protein-1. J Biol Chem 2004;279:980–6.

[32] Bourd-Boittin K, Fridman R, Fanchon S, et al. Matrix metalloproteinase inhibition impairs the processing, formation and mineralization of dental tissues during mouse molar development. Exp Cell Res 2005;304:493–505.

[33] Fanchon S, Bourd K, Septier D, et al. Involvement of matrix metalloproteinases in the onset of dentin mineralization. Eur J Oral Sci 2004;112:171–6.

[34] Ohshima H. Ultrastructural changes in odontoblasts and pulp capillaries following cavity preparation in rat molars. Arch Histol Cytol 1990;53:423–38.

[35] Six N, Lasfargues J-J, Goldberg M. In vivo study off the pulp reaction to Fuji IX, a glass ionomer cement. J Dent 2000;28:413–22.

[36] Decup F, Six N, Palmier B, et al. Bone sialoprotein-induced reparative dentinogenesis in the pulp of rat's molar. Clin Oral Invest 2000;4:110–9.

[37] Wang J, Glimcher MJ, Mah J, et al. Expression of bone microsomal casein kinase II, bone sialoprotein, and osteopontin during the repair of calvaria defects. Bone 1998;22:621–8.

[38] Wang J, Glimcher MJ. Characterization of matrix-induced osteogenesis in rat calvarial bone defects: I. Differences in the cellular response to demineralized bone matrix implanted in calvarial defects and in subcutaneous sites. Calcif Tissue Int 1999;65:156–65.

[39] Wang J, Glimcher MJ. Characterization of matrix-induced osteogenesis in rat calvarial bone defects: II Origins of bone-forming cells. Calcif Tissue Int 1999;65:486–93.

[40] Hunter GK, Goldberg HA. Modulation of crystal formation by bone phosphoprotein: role of glutamic acid-rich sequences in the nucleation of hydroxyapatite by bone sialoprotein. Biochem J 1994;302:175–9.

[41] Fujisawa R, Kuboki Y. Affinity of bone sialoprotein and several other bone and dnetin acidic proteins to collagen fibrils. Calcif Tissue Int 1992;51:438–42.

[42] Chen J, Shapiro HS, Sodek J. Developmental expression of bone sialoprotein mRNA in rat mineralized connective tissues. J Bone Miner Res 1992;7:987–97.

[43] Chen J, McCullogh CAG, Sodek J. Bone sialoprotein in developing porcine dental tissues: cellular expression and comparison of tissue localization with osteopontin and osteonectin. Arch Oral Biol 1993;38:241–9.

[44] Rutherford B, Fitzgerald M. A new biological approach to vital pulp therapy. Crit Rev Oral Biol Med 1995;6:218–29.

[45] MacDougall M, Simmons D, Gu TT, et al. MEPE/OF45, a new dentin/bone matrix protein and candidate gene for dentin diseases mapping to chromosome 4q21. Connect Tissue Res 2002;43:320–30.

[46] Argiro L, Desbarats M, Glorieux FH, et al. Mepe, the gene encoding a tumor-secreted protein in oncogenic hypophosphatemic osteomalacia, is expressed in bone. Genomics 2001;74: 342–51.

[47] Rowe PS, Kumagai Y, Gutierrez G, et al. MEPE has the properties of an osteoblastic phosphatonin and minhibin. Bone 2004;34:303–19.

[48] Rowe PSH. The wrickkened pathway of FGF23, MEPE and Phex. Crit Rev Oral Biol Med 2004;15:264–81.

[49] Liu H, Li W, Gao C, et al. Dentonin, a fragment of MEPE, enhanced dental pulp stem cell proliferation. J Dent Res 2004;83:496–9.

[50] Amar S, Sires B, Sabsay B, et al. The isolation and partial characterization of a rat incisor dentin matrix polypeptide with in vitro chondrogenic activity. J Biol Chem 1991;266: 8609–18.

[51] Nebgen DR, Inoue H, Sabsay B, et al. Identification of the chondrogenic-inducing activity from bovine dentin (bCIA) as a low-molecular-mass amelogenin polypetide. J Dent Res 1999;78:1484–94.

[52] Veis A, Tompkins K, Alvares K, et al. Specific amelogenin gene splice products have signaling effects on cell in culture and implant in vivo. J Biol Chem 2000;275:41263–72.

[53] Goldberg M, Lacerda-Pinheiro S, Chardin H, et al. Implantation of two low molecular weight amelogenins (A + 4 and A−4) in the pulp of rat's maxillary molars and in an oral mucosa ectopic site. In: Landis W, Sodek J, co-chairs. Proceedings of the Eighth International Conference on the Chemistry and Biology of Mineralized Tissues (2004). p. 115–7.

[54] Wurst T, Krüger A, Christersson C, et al. A new protein expressed in bone marrow cells and osteoblasts with implication in osteoblast recruitment. Exp Cell Res 2001;263:236–42.

[55] Krüger A, Ellerstrtöm C, Lundmark C, et al. RP59, a marker for osteoblast recruitment, is alos detected in primitive mesenchymal cells, erythroid cells, and megacaryocytes. Dev Dyn 2002;223:414–8.

[56] Priam F, Ronco V, Locker M, et al. New cellular models for tracking the odontoblast phenotype. Arch Oral Biol 2005;50:271–7.

[57] Lacerda-Pinheiro S, Jegat N, Septier D, et al. Early in vivo and in vitro effects of amelogenin gene splice products on pulp cells. Eur J Oral Sci, in press.

[58] Peister A, Mellad JA, Larson BL, et al. Adult stem cells from bone marrow (MSCs) isolated from different strains of inbred mice vary in surface epitopes, rates of proliferation, and differentiation potential. Blood 2004;103:1662–8.

[59] Kuwana M, Okazaki Y, Kodama H, et al. Human circulating CD14 + monocytes as source of progenitors that exhibit mesenchymal cell differentiation. J Leukoc Biol 2003;74:833–45.

ELSEVIER
SAUNDERS

Dent Clin N Am 50 (2006) 299–315

The Outlook for Implants and Endodontics: A Review of the Tissue Engineering Strategies to Create Replacement Teeth for Patients

Peter E. Murray, PhD*, Franklin García-Godoy, DDS, MS

College of Dental Medicine, Nova Southeastern University, 3200 South University Drive, Fort Lauderdale, FL 33328, USA

Pulpal regeneration after tooth injury is not easy to accomplish, which is why the infected pulp requires tooth extraction or root canal therapy. Otherwise, more serious complications, such as periapical lesions, can occur [1]. In a few cases, partial pulpotomy, sometimes called Cvek pulpotomy [2], is the treatment of choice for injured permanent incisor teeth with exposed vital pulp tissue and immature apices [3]. This treatment preserves pulpal function and allows continued root development.

The healing of severely damaged teeth is difficult to accomplish [4]. The major problem seems to be the lack of ability of the dental pulp to regenerate its cell populations and mineralized structures after injury or infection. The loss or fracture of tooth dentin may expose the pulp tissue during operative dental treatment, because of accidental injury, or as a result of caries decay. The placement of a dental material in contact with exposed pulp tissue to restore the tooth structure is called direct pulp capping, and the placement of a dental material without any pulp contact is called indirect pulp capping. The prognosis of direct pulp capped teeth is much reduced in comparison with indirect pulp capped teeth. The success of direct pulp capping treatment is 37% after 5 years and 13% after 10 years [5], which compares with an 86% rate of success for indirect pulp capped teeth over 10 years [6]. Because of this low rate of treatment success, most dentists immediately

This work was supported by a grant from the American Association of Endodontists Foundation.

* Corresponding author.

E-mail address: petemurr@nsu.nova.edu (P.E. Murray).

refer patients for pulpotomy of part or all of the pulp tissue or extraction of the tooth [7]. This approach is one reason for the 21 million teeth that develop symptoms requiring endodontic therapy and the uncounted millions of teeth that are extracted every year in the United States [8]. One fourth of all Americans aged 65 to 74 have had all their teeth extracted. There seems to be a large variation between socioeconomic groups and states. Hawaii has the lowest rate of tooth extraction (13.9%) and West Virginia has the highest (47%) [9]. After tooth extraction, patients have the option of wearing artificial tooth implants or dentures. Currently, 45 million Americans wear dentures; one fourth are dissatisfied with these artificial teeth [9]. Each year, more than $60 billion are spent on professional dental treatments in the United States. The numbers and types of dental treatments are shown in Table 1.

Many aspects of endodontic therapy have proved to be controversial. A recent meta-analysis of the success rate for single versus multiple visit endodontic treatment found no significant difference in the success rate of teeth healing after apical periodontitis [10]. A survey of 350 endodontic treated teeth over 5 years reported that specialist endodontists can accomplish a treatment success rate of 98.1% compared with general dentists, who can accomplish a success rate of 89.7% [11]. The success rate of more than 85% for endodontically treated teeth seems to be supported by the dental literature [12–14]. It should be noted, however, that there is a general lack of information on long-term treatment success and that variations in the preoperative periapical status and the apical limit of the obturation may influence strongly the longevity of treatment [15].

During the last two decades, dental implants have become increasingly used as an alternative to conventional removable dentures. Some clinical studies have indicated that implant therapy has a favorable long-term prognosis [16]. The success rate of dental implants is approximately 90% [17,18]. The high clinical survival rate even in partially edentulous patients has led to a widespread acceptance and use of oral implants [19]. Problems do occur, however. Factors such as bone quality, surgical trauma, and bacterial contamination during implant surgery have been associated with early failures [20]. Overload, defined as a situation in which the functional load applied to the implants exceeds the capacity of the bone implant interface to withstand

Table 1
Numbers of dental treatments in the United States in millions per year

Dental treatments	Millions/y
Dental restorative treatments	300
Periodontal therapies	80
Endodontics (root canal therapies)	21
Cleft palate and birth defect surgery	0.25
Craniofacial trauma victims who require surgery	0.15
Cancer	0.03
Implants	0.1+

Stem cell therapies may impact all these dental treatments in the future.

it, is another possible cause of implant failure once the prosthesis is installed. Factors associated with late failures of implants are less well understood and seem to be related to the peri-implant environment and host parameters [21].

The 90% treatment success rates reported in the literature are a direct result of the dental profession continuing to improve the standard and quality of care provided to patients. To replace existing dental treatments, any new therapy must be proved to be more successful. The high success rates of existing dental therapies must be matched or exceeded by tissue engineering therapies if they are to be used successfully by the dental profession. This presents a formidable goal and barrier to the introduction of dental therapies that use tissue engineering approaches to regenerate diseased, lost, and missing teeth.

Odontoblasts and dentinogenesis

The successful resolution of restorative treatments depends on harnessing and using the natural repair responses of the pulpal cell populations, especially odontoblasts [22]. Odontoblasts are highly differentiated postmitotic cells that regulate dentin synthesis, secretion, and mineralization throughout life [23]. The other pulpal cell populations that occupy the subodontoblast layer and the pulp core are important in supporting dentinogenesis but do not seem to play a direct role in the secretion of dentin matrix [24]. The maintenance and repair of dentin are accomplished by the secretory activity of the odontoblast cells [25]. The odontoblasts are located peripherally around the pulp with their cellular process transversing dentin, and these cells have been demonstrated to detect and respond to dentin injury after caries and restorative dental procedures [26–31]. The rate of dentin secretion by odontoblasts has been observed to vary according to the chronology and circumstances of its secretion. Dentin can be classified as primary, secondary, or tertiary in origin. In humans, primary dentin is secreted at a rate of approximately 4 μm/d during tooth development until the completion of root formation [32]. Thereafter, physiologic secondary dentin is laid down at a reducing rate of approximately 0.5 μm/d along the pulp-dentin border throughout life [33,34]. Essentially, the odontoblasts go into a resting state after primary dentinogenesis, and the limited rate of secondary dentin formation over several decades represents a basal level of activity. If the dentin should become damaged, however, the synthesis and secretion of dentin are upregulated by the underlying odontoblasts to provide pulp protection. The increase in dentin secretion is called tertiary dentinogenesis because it is a dentin regenerative response by the odontoblasts. The histology of the pulp-dentin complex of teeth is shown in Fig. 1.

Tertiary dentinogenesis

The process of tertiary dentin secretion can be classified as reactionary in origin, depending on the severity of the initiating response and the

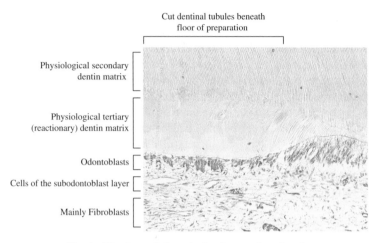

Cut dentinal tubules beneath
floor of preparation

Physiological secondary
dentin matrix

Physiological tertiary
(reactionary) dentin matrix

Odontoblasts

Cells of the subodontoblast layer

Mainly Fibroblasts

Fig. 1. Histology of the pulp-dentin complex of teeth.

conditions under which the dentin matrix was secreted [35–37]. The secretion of reactionary dentin is the main postoperative odontoblast repair response to an unexposed cavity restoration that has been cut carefully into the dentin of a tooth [38]. The rate at which reactionary dentin has been estimated to be laid down is 1.5 μm/d [39]. This rate is approximately three times the rate of normal secondary dentin mineralization. The secretion of reactionary dentin is initiated in response to environmental and accidental events, such as caries, attrition, abrasion, erosion, accidental trauma, and restorative dentistry. Sources of injury associated with restorative procedures have included acid etching of the cavity wall [40], presence of bacteria [41–43], method of placement of the restorative material [35,44], desiccation [45], pulpal inflammation relating to the remaining dentin thickness [46,47], chemical irritants [48], restoration material toxicity [49], and restoration material temperature [50,51]. Odontoblast survival is a multifactorial process and these factors may play a role individually or cumulatively in the degree of injury to the odontoblasts. If odontoblasts are not injured or are injured slightly, then no increase in dentinogenesis is likely to be observed in teeth. After more severe injury, some reactionary dentin deposition may be observed to repair lost or injured secondary dentin matrix. The secretion of reactionary dentin is proportional to the degree of injury to the pulp dentin tissue and the number of surviving functional odontoblasts [52].

If the odontoblasts are destroyed because of dentin injury or pulp exposure, then no reactionary dentin repair can be accomplished because no functional secretory odontoblast cells remain. Instead, pulp dentin repair is accomplished by an entirely different form of tertiary dentin called reparative dentinogenesis [53]. The reparative form of tertiary dentinogenesis is a much more complex biologic process than the reactionary type, because it involves the differentiation, proliferation, and migration of a new cell population to replace the odontoblasts that were destroyed. An important factor that influences the severity of pulp dentin injury, the survival of odontoblasts, and their secretion of tertiary dentin is the remaining dentin thickness of dental preparations [54]. A schematic diagram of the relationship between remaining dentin thickness as the source of injury and the pulp healing response is shown in Fig. 2.

Reparative dentinogenesis

The dental pulp has a well-documented ability to form hard tissue barriers called reparative dentin after direct pulp capping or pulpotomy. If the reparative dentinogenesis forms across the wound site of a pulp exposure, it is called a dentin bridge (henceforth called a reparative dentin bridge) [55,56]. Ideally, a reparative dentin bridge establishes complete dentinal closure of the pulpal tissue; its presence after capping of the pulp exposure is observed in 90% of human pulps and is considered to be a sign of successful healing [4]. The structure of reparative dentin bridge can resemble tubular physiologic secondary dentin matrix, attubular osteodentin, or

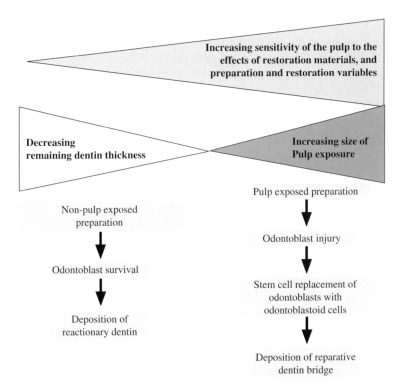

Fig. 2. Model of human pulp healing activity in response to the remaining dentin thickness of dental preparations.

globular fibrodentin. Fibrodentin formed as an intermediate matrix zone during the wound-healing process has been suggested for the initiation of reparative dentin bridge formation [26]. The observations of different types of reparative dentin bridge suggest that it is the culmination of a multistage regenerative process. The variable quality in reparative structure can influence dentin permeability in the wound region. Dentin permeability is the most important factor that determines pulp reactions to caries, operative procedures, and localized lesions [57]. A high permeability allows toxic substances from materials and bacteria leakage to reach the pulp easily [58], and they can act as irritants if their concentration reaches an inflammatory threshold [59]. The barrier properties of the reparative dentin bridge are advantageous for preserving the vitality of the pulp tissues, which explains the widespread interest in the process of reparative dentinogenesis and the number of investigations that assess the role of pulp dentin injury and restorative materials. Tooth dentin and reparative dentin bridge provide better protection for the pulp tissue than any restorative material [60]. The ability of the reparative dentin bridge to seal the site of tooth injury depends on the activity of the dental pulp stem cells (Fig. 3).

Source of pulp stem cells

Much attention has focused on the origin of the odontoblastoid cells that secrete the matrix for reparative dentin bridge. After severe pulp damage or mechanical or caries exposure, the odontoblasts are often irreversibly injured beneath the wound site [54]. Odontoblasts are postmitotic terminally differentiated cells and cannot proliferate to replace subjacent irreversibly injured odontoblasts [61]. The source of the odontoblastoid cells that replace

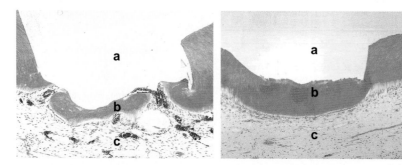

Fig. 3. Reparative dentin bridge formation by pulp stem cells. The histology of reparative dentin bridging is shown in two different teeth after direct pulp exposure. The dentin bridge formed on the right side is complete. Note the site of pulp exposure (*a*), the dentin bridge (*b*), and pulp tissue (*c*). (*Left*) The gaps in the dentin bridge probably were caused by a failure of the pulp stem cells to reach some parts of the site of injury and secrete tertiary dentin. In this case, blood clots may have been responsible. (*Right*) The complete formation of the dentin bridge suggests that the pulp stem cells were able to align across the site of pulp exposure. The addition of pulp stem cells may improve the quality of pulp repair.

the odontoblasts and secrete reparative dentin bridges has proved to be controversial. Initially, the replacement of irreversibly injured odontoblasts by predetermined odontoblastoid cells that do not replicate their DNA after induction was suggested. Researchers proposed that the cells within the sub-odontoblast cell-rich layer or zone of Hohl adjacent to the odontoblasts differentiate into odontoblastoids [62]. The purpose of these cells seems to be limited to an odontoblast supporting role, however, because the survival of these cells was linked to the survival of the odontoblasts, and no proliferative or regenerative activity was observed. The use of tritiated thymidine to study cellular division in the pulp by autoradiography after damage [63] revealed a peak in fibroblast activity close to the exposure site approximately 4 days after successful pulp capping of monkey teeth [64].

An additional autoradiographic study of dentin bridge formation in monkey teeth after calcium hydroxide direct pulp capping for up to 12 days revealed differences in the cellular labeling depending on the location of the wound site [65]. Labeling of specific cells among the fibroblasts and perivascular cells shifted from low to high over time if the exposure was limited to the odontoblastic layer and the cell-free zone, whereas labeling changed from high to low if the exposure was deep into the pulpal tissue. More cells were labeled close to the reparative dentin bridge than in the pulp core. The autoradiographic findings did not show any labeling in the existing odontoblast layer or in a specific pulp location. The findings provided support for the theory that the progenitor stem cells for the odontoblastoid cells are resident undifferentiated mesenchymal cells [63]. The origins of these cells may be related to the primary odontoblasts, because during tooth development, only the neural crest–derived cell population of the dental papilla is able to respond specifically to the basement membrane–mediated inductive signal for odontoblast differentiation [66,67]. The ability of young and old teeth to respond to injury by induction of reparative dentinogenesis suggests that a similar population of competent progenitor cells still may exist within the dental pulp, which can later differentiate into odontoblastoid cells. The debate on the nature of the precursor stem cells giving rise to the odontoblastoids and questions concerning the heterogeneity of the dental pulp population in adult teeth remain to be resolved [68,69].

Stem cells are defined by their capacity for asymmetric division, wherein a single cell division can give rise to one cell identical to the mother cell, a new stem cell, and another more differentiated cell [70]. The latter can be predetermined if it arises from a committed stem cell, whereas pluripotential stem cells can give rise to diverse progeny. Committed stem cells arise from these pluripotential stem cells, such as the adult mesenchymal stem cell or the embryonic stem cell. Although in adults, mesenchymal stem cells reside in hematopoietic tissue, committed stem cells often are located in the deep layers of tissues, where they are positioned to restore continuously the outer tissue cells lost during aging or mobilize rapidly to restore function after disease or trauma [71]. Mesenchymal stem cells may have the potential to regenerate diseased, lost, and missing human dental structures [72]. A schematic representation of the lifecycle and activity of dental pulp stem cells is shown in Fig. 4.

Molecular regulation of dental pulp stem cell migration

Directional migration of stem cells is necessary for embryonic development and homeostatic maintenance and repair of injured organs and tissues in adults [73]. In the absence of migration, the contribution of stem cells to the development of functional organs and tissues would not be possible, because all stem cells must migrate to sites at which they are required to function. We have studied the molecular regulation of dental pulp stem cells and have found some similarities to the mechanisms of migration in other cell types. The Rho family of GTPases constitutes a family of intracellular messengers that are regulated by their location and state of activation. They seem to exert important influences in almost all functions of the stem cell, including adherence and migration [74]. Rho seems to exert important effects on cellular contraction and detachment, whereas Rac exerts effects needed for directed migration of polarized cells. Cdc42 activates many of the same receptors as Rac, but its effects seem limited to those involving cellular morphology and lamillopodia development. Preliminary studies have demonstrated Rac as being at the leading edge of migrating cells where Rho is either inactivated or disintegrated. Conversely, at the tail edge of migrating stem cells, activated Rho associates with its effector Rho kinase. The

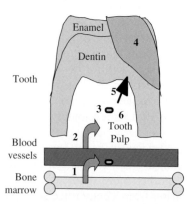

Fig. 4. Adult stem cell life cycle and activity. The sequence of the life cycle of adult stem activity is as follows: (*1*) Pluripotential mesenchymal stem cells reside in bone marrow. (*2*) These cells are mobilized to the circulation in response to specific factors generated during injury or infection. They localize to the site where needed by chemotactic migration through local tissue and differentiate into committed stem cells (*3*). In teeth they are known as pulp stem cells. (*4*) Tooth damage stimulates pulp stem cell migration and differentiation (*5*), which results in restoration of tooth structure, whereas asymmetric cell division maintains the pulp stem cell population (*6*).

effector or Rac that leads to actin development and migration is not clear but seems to be a unique enzyme, Pak-1 [75].

The kinase activity of Pak-1 is enhanced when it engages Rac in its GTP "activated" form. The targets for the enzyme that are essential for mobility are not clear, but myosin kinases activated by P13 kinase products, the stress kinase p38, and cell contractibility have been implicated. In the nucleus, the tumor suppressor protein p27 kip binds with its amino terminal region (N) to complexes of cyclins and cyclin-dependent kinases (CDKs) to inhibit cell proliferation. When phosphorylated, p27 kip1 might move into the cytoplasm, where, as shown by Besson and colleagues [76], it binds through its carboxy terminus to RhoA and interfaces with RhoA activation by guanine-nucleotide-exchange factors. RhoA, Cdc42, and Rac regulate the cytoskeletal changes required for cell migration. Cdc42 and Rac work mainly at the front of polarized cells and regulate the actin-driven protrusion and the formation of new adhesions required for forward movement. RhoA, through the Rho-associated kinase (ROCK) protein, works mainly at the rear and determines (among other processes) the turnover of adhesive sites, known as focal adhesions and rear retraction. By interfering with RhoA activation, focal adhesion kinase (FAK) inhibits or promotes cell migration, depending on the cell type. The migration of dental pulp stem cells seems to be controlled by a balance in Rac/Rho-kinase activation. When Rac is activated the cell migrates forward; when Rho-kinase is activated the cell remains fixed in position. Our hypotheses for the signaling pathways between the proteins involved in cell migration are summarized in Fig. 5. These proteins are useful targets for developing drugs to control stem cell migration as part of tissue engineering therapies.

Stem cell therapy

Stem cell therapy is one of the most promising areas of tissue engineering because the transplantation of materials that contain pulp stem cells grown in the laboratory provides an excellent inductive means to regenerate new tooth tissues. The transplantation of odontoblastoid stem cells into teeth to accomplish regeneration removes the problems of delivering growth factors and genes into host target cells and waiting for the target cells to differentiate, proliferate, and migrate to sites of injury before the reparative activity can commence. These considerations are important because pulp tissue replacement must be almost immediate to begin the regeneration of tooth tissues before the restorative treatment irreversibly fails. The use of cultured cells derived from adult human pulp tissue to regenerate lost cell populations eliminates the ethical drawbacks associated with fetal stem cell therapy. Because of ethical and legal restrictions associated with fetal human pulp stem cells, attention has focused on the xenotransplantation of human tissues into animals. Recently researchers called for a moratorium on research using xenographs because of the health hazards that this therapy presents to humans [77].

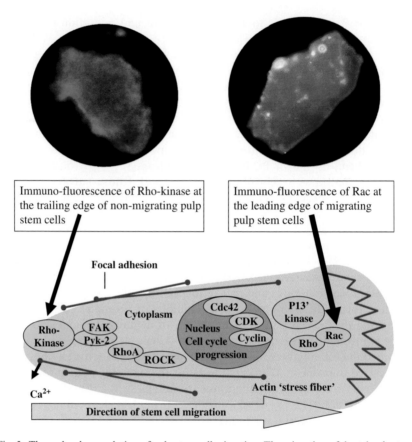

Fig. 5. The molecular regulation of pulp stem cell migration. The migration of dental pulp stem cells seems to be controlled by a balance in the Rac/Rho-kinase activation. When Rac is activated, the cell migrates forward. When Rho-kinase is activated, the cell remains fixed in position. The signaling pathways between Rac and Rho-kinase are shown here.

Recent studies focused on evaluating the use of human odontoblastoid stem cell transplantation for regenerating oral tissues in conjunction with in vitro tissue engineering to produce regenerative biomimetic materials.

Stem cell engineering of biomimetic materials

The regeneration of decayed or lost tooth tissue is problematic. No restorative material exists that can be placed into a tooth provides better protection for pulp tissue than dentin [78]. Any injury to the dentin pulp complex can trigger inflammatory cell activity [79]. These inflammatory reactions can injure the pulpal cell populations and lead to complications [80]. If unchecked, severe inflammatory activity often can progress to total pulp necrosis and lesion development followed by local bone destruction [81].

Observations of the low success rates of some types of restorative materials and how they contribute to postoperative complications, such as hypersensitivity, pulp inflammation [82], and treatment failure, have stimulated interest in the transplantation of natural tooth substance, which has been grown using in vitro culture. Few restorative materials share the same physical or chemical characteristics of the natural tooth, which may explain why a high proportion of cavity restorations fail mechanically. Resin-modified glass ionomer is a common restorative material [83]; however, surveys show that more than 50% of these restorations require replacement because of mechanical failure [84,85]. Few restorative materials share the appearance of tooth aesthetics, although resin composite materials can be color matched [86]. These results contrast with the use of tooth tissue, which shares the same chemical, physical, and aesthetic properties of natural teeth. These properties are ideal for restoring damaged tooth surfaces because abrasion, erosion, attrition, and tooth wear remain prevalent [87]. Porcelain veneers are often placed for aesthetic purposes, but the low success rates and longevity of this treatment would make the immediate replacement of lost tooth surfaces with synthetically mineralized tooth tissues a welcome advance in restorative dentistry [88].

Harvesting teeth created by tissue engineering

The ability to create in the laboratory teeth that can be harvested and implanted into patients to restore extracted or lost teeth long has been a goal for dental research [89,90]. The characterization of dental mesenchymal differentiation into pulp, dentin, and enamel has highlighted some developmental processes that may be used by tissue engineering therapies to create synthetic teeth [35,91–94]. The growth and formation of new teeth has been partially successful, because only small parts of tooth structures have been created and all of the approaches used existing developmental tooth structures as a template [95–97]. The development of tissue engineering science recently allowed new tissues, such as small intestine tissue, to be created after seeding stem cells onto biodegradable polymer scaffolds [98]. The use of this tissue engineering technique has allowed the formation of tooth crowns from stem cells taken from porcine third molars [99]. After the cell/polymer constructs have been formed using in vitro tissue culture, they are implanted into a suitable host animal to provide a vascular blood supply to support the growth and development of higher ordered tissue structures [100].

Adult human pulp stem cells have not yet used these techniques to create human teeth by tissue engineering, however. We propose that the future creation of replacement teeth for patients involve a chair-side technology with the following process: The first step is to create a computer-aided biomodel of the oral cavity and analyze the aesthetics of existing teeth. The second step is to use a database of tooth sizes, shapes, and aesthetics as a blueprint for designing a replacement tooth. The third step is to biomanufacture the tooth using a scaffold and three-dimensional cell pattern printing and deposition methods. Slabs of biosynthetic enamel and dentin are cut into the shape of the tooth. The forth step is to implant the tooth surgically into the patient and reconnect blood flow, nerves, and periodontal ligaments. This process for the tissue engineering of a replacement tooth is shown in Fig. 6. Much of this technology already exists or is close to development, and the goal for dental researchers is to put the technology together and make it work reliably.

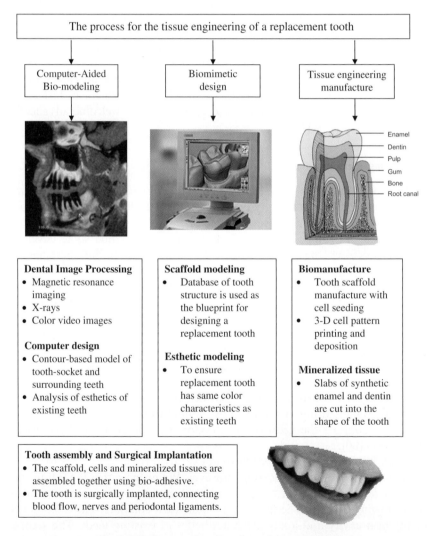

Fig. 6. The tissue engineering of a replacement tooth.

Significance of tissue engineering therapy

An increase in the success of restorative dental treatment will transform completely the economics of oral health in the United States. Every year it is estimated that $60 billion are spent on dental expenditure [101]; $5 billion per year has been saved, mostly because of preventive dentistry [102]. Total expenditure continues to increase every year, however. Because two thirds of all restorative dentistry cases involve the replacement of failed treatments, a tremendous potential remains for improvement [81,82]. Even a small percentage of increase in the ability to preserve severely injured teeth could cut dental expenditure dramatically by reducing the number of patients who require dentures or tooth implants. Forty-five million Americans wear dentures, and at least one fourth are dissatisfied with these artificial teeth [9]. Although there always has been a need to minimize the number of teeth that are extracted, the limited ability of conventional restorative treatments to regenerate teeth has prevented dentists from saving many diseased and damaged teeth from extraction. The introduction of stem cell–based therapies means that more teeth may be saved, which could reduce dramatically the numbers of Americans who must wear dentures or care for their artificial tooth implants. This progress will improve the quality of life for millions of ordinary people.

References

[1] Jansson L, Ehnevid H, Lindskog S, et al. Development of periapical lesions. Swed Dent J 1993;17(3):85–93.
[2] Cvek M. A clinical report on partial pulpotomy and capping with calcium hydroxide in permanent incisors with complicated crown fracture. J Endod 1978;4(8):232–7.
[3] Sari S. Cvek pulpotomy: report of a case with five-year follow-up. ASDC J Dent Child 2002; 69(1):27–30.
[4] Baume LJ, Holtz L. Long term clinical assessment of direct pulp capping. Int Dent J 1981; 31(4):251–60.
[5] Barthel CR, Rosenkranz B, Leuenberg A, et al. Pulp capping of carious exposures: treatment outcome after 5 and 10 years: a retrospective study. J Endod 2000;26(9):525–8.
[6] Mertz-Fairhurst EJ, Curtis JW, Ergle JW, et al. Ultraconservative and cariostatic sealed restorations: results at year 10. J Am Dent Assoc 1998;129(1):55–66.
[7] Ranly DM, Garcia-Godoy F. Current and potential pulp therapies for primary and young permanent teeth. J Dent 2000;28(3):153–61.
[8] Stanley HR. Pulp capping: conserving the dental pulp. Can it be done? Is it worth it? Oral Surg Oral Med Oral Pathol 1989;68(5):628–39.
[9] Lechner SK, Roessler D. Strategies for complete denture success: beyond technical excellence. Compend Contin Educ Dent 2001;22(7):553–9.
[10] Sathorn C, Parashos P, Messer HH. Effectiveness of single- versus multiple-visit endodontic treatment of teeth with apical periodontitis: a systematic review and meta-analysis. Int Endod J 2005;38(6):347–55.
[11] Alley BS, Kitchens GG, Alley LW, et al. A comparison of survival of teeth following endodontic treatment performed by general dentists or by specialists. Oral Surg Oral Med Oral Pathol Oral Radiol Endod 2004;98(1):115–8.

[12] Siqueira JF Jr. Strategies to treat infected root canals. J Calif Dent Assoc 2001;29(12): 825–37.

[13] Peak JD. The success of endodontic treatment in general dental practice: a retrospective clinical and radiographic study. Prim Dent Care 1994;1(1):9–13.

[14] Teo CS, Chan NC, Lim SS. Success rate in endodontic therapy: a retrospective study. Part I. Dent J Malays 1986;9(1):7–10.

[15] Basmadjian-Charles CL, Farge P, Bourgeois DM, et al. Factors influencing the long-term results of endodontic treatment: a review of the literature. Int Dent J 2002;52(2):81–6.

[16] Berglundh T, Persson L, Klinge B. A systematic review of the incidence of biological and technical complications in implant dentistry reported in prospective longitudinal studies of at least 5 years. J Clin Periodontol 2002;29(3):197–212.

[17] Del Fabbro M, Testori T, Francetti L, et al. Systematic review of survival rates for implants placed in the grafted maxillary sinus. Int J Periodontics Restorative Dent 2004;24(6):565–77.

[18] Sweeney IP, Ferguson JW, Heggie AA, et al. Treatment outcomes for adolescent ectodermal dysplasia patients treated with dental implants. Int J Paediatr Dent 2005;15(4):241–8.

[19] Van der Weijden GA, van Bemmel KM, Renvert S. Implant therapy in partially edentulous, periodontally compromised patients: a review. J Clin Periodontol 2005;32(5):506–11.

[20] Esposito M, Coulthard P, Thomsen P, et al. The role of implant surface modifications, shape and material on the success of osseointegrated dental implants: a Cochrane systematic review. Eur J Prosthodont Restor Dent 2005;13(1):15–31.

[21] Quirynen M, De Soete M, van Steenberghe D. Infectious risks for oral implants: a review of the literature. Clin Oral Implants Res 2002;13(1):1–19.

[22] Murray PE, Smith AJ. Saving pulps: a biological basis. An overview. Prim Dent Care 2002; 9(1):21–6.

[23] Murray PE, Stanley HR, Matthews JB, et al. Age-related odontometric changes of human teeth. Oral Surg Oral Med Oral Pathol 2002;93(4):474–82.

[24] Linde A. The extracellular matrix of the dental pulp and dentin. J Dent Res 1985;64(Spec Iss):523–9.

[25] Stanley HR, Periera JC, Speigel E, et al. The detection and prevalence of reactive, reparative dentin and dead tracts beneath various types of dental lesions according to tooth surface and age. J Oral Pathol 1983;12(4):257–89.

[26] Baume LJ. Monographs in oral science. Basel (Switzerland): Karger; 1980.

[27] Stanley HR. Human pulp response to restorative dental procedures. Gainesville (FL): Sorter Printing Co.; 1981.

[28] Cox CF, White KC, Ramus DL, et al. Reparative dentin: factors affecting its deposition. Quintess Int 1992;23(4):257–70.

[29] Smith AJ, Tobias RS, Cassidy N, et al. Odontoblast stimulation of ferrets by dentin matrix components. Arch Oral Biol 1994;39(1):13–22.

[30] Robertson A, Lundgren T, Andreason JO, et al. Pulp calcifications in traumatized primary incisors: a morphological and inductive analysis study. Eur J Oral Sci 1997;105(3):196–206.

[31] About I, Laurent-Maquin D, Lendahl U, et al. Nestin expression in embryonic and adult teeth under normal and physiological conditions. Am J Pathol 2000;157(1):287–95.

[32] Kawasaki K, Tanaka S, Ishikawa T. On the daily incremental lines in human dentine. Arch Oral Biol 1979;24(12):939–43.

[33] Morse DR. Age-related changes of the dental pulp complex and their relationship to systemic ageing. Oral Surg Oral Med Oral Pathol 1991;72(6):721–45.

[34] Solheim T. Amount of secondary dentin as an indicator of age. Scand J Dent Res 1992; 100(4):193–9.

[35] Linde A, Goldberg M. Dentinogenesis. Crit Rev Oral Biol Med 1993;4(5):679–728.

[36] Linde A, Lundgren T. From serum to the mineral phase: the role of the odontoblast in calcium transport and mineral formation. Int J Dev Biol 1995;39(1):213–22.

[37] Smith AJ, Cassidy N, Perry H, et al. Reactionary dentinogenesis. Int J Dev Biol 1995;39(1): 273–80.

[38] Murray PE, About I, Lumley PJ, et al. Postoperative pulpal and repair responses. J Am Dent Assoc 2000;131(3):321–9.

[39] Stanley HR, White CL, McCray L. The rate of tertiary (reparative) dentin formation in the human tooth. Oral Surg Oral Med Oral Pathol 1966;21(2):180–9.

[40] Gwinnet AJ, Tay F. Early or intermediate response of the human pulp to acid etch technique in vivo. Am J Dent 1998;11(Spec Iss):S35–44.

[41] Bergenholtz G. Effect of bacterial products on inflammatory reactions in the dental pulp. Scand J Dent Res 1977;85(2):122–9.

[42] Chong BS, Pitt Ford TR, Kariyawasam SP. Short-term tissue response to potential root-end filling materials in infected root canals. Int Endod J 1997;30(4):240–9.

[43] Camps J, Dejou J, Remusat M, et al. Factors influencing pulpal response to cavity restorations. Dent Mat 2000;16(6):432–40.

[44] Sigurdsson A, Stancill R, Madison S. Intracanal placement of Ca(OH)2: a comparison of techniques. J Endod 1992;18(8):367–70.

[45] Brannstrom M. Communication between the oral cavity and the dental pulp associated with restorative treatment. Operat Dent 1984;9(2):57–68.

[46] Tobias RS, Plant CG, Browne RM. Reduction in pulpal inflammation beneath surface-sealed silicates. Int Endod J 1982;15(4):173–80.

[47] Sazak S, Gunday M, Alatli C. Effect of calcium hydroxide and combinations of ledermix and calcium hydroxide on inflamed pulp in dogs' teeth. J Endod 1996;22(9):447–9.

[48] Kawasaki K, Ruben J, Stokroos I, et al. The remineralization of EDTA-treated human dentine. Caries Res 1999;33(4):275–80.

[49] Cox CF. Microleakage related to restorative procedures. Proc Finn Dent Soc 1992; 88(Suppl 1):83–93.

[50] Stewart G, Bachman T, Hatton J. Temperature rise due to finishing of direct restorative materials. Am J Dent 1991;4(1):23–8.

[51] Anil N, Keyf F. Temperature change in the pulp chamber during the application of heat to composite and amalgam cores and its returning time to oral heat. Int Dent J 1996;46(4): 362–6.

[52] Murray PE, About I, Franquin JC, et al. Restorative pulpal and repair responses. J Am Dent Assoc 2001;132(4):482–91 Erratum in J Am Dent Assoc 2001;132(8):1095.

[53] Smith AJ, Cassidy N, Perry H, et al. Reactionary dentinogenesis. Int J Dev Biol 1995;39(1): 273–80.

[54] Murray PE, About I, Lumley PJ, et al. Cavity remaining dentin thickness and pulpal activity. Am J Dent 2002;15(1):41–6.

[55] Schröder U. Effects of calcium hydroxide-containing pulp-capping agents on pulp cell migration, proliferation, and differentiation. J Dent Res 1985;64(Spec Iss):541–8.

[56] Tziafas D. Mechanisms controlling secondary initiation of dentinogenesis: a review. Int Endod J 1994;27(2):61–74.

[57] Mjor IA. Dentin and pulp: reaction patterns in human teeth. Boca Raton (FL): CRC Press; 1983.

[58] Pashley DH. Mechanisms of dentin sensitivity. Dent Clin N Am 1990;34(3):449–73.

[59] Pashley DH. Dentin permeability: theory and practice. In: Spangberg L, editor. Experimental endodontics. Boca Raton (FL): CRC Press; 1989. p. 19–49.

[60] Smith AJ, Sloan AJ, Matthews JB, et al. Reparative processes in dentine and pulp. In: Addy M, Embery G, Edgar WM, editors. Tooth wear and sensitivity. London: Martin-Dunitz; 2000. p. 53–66.

[61] Murray PE, Lumley PJ, Ross HF, et al. Tooth slice organ culture for cytotoxicity assessment of dental materials. Biomaterials 2000;21(16):1711–21.

[62] Höhl E. Beitrag zur histologie der pulpa und des dentins. Archives Anatomic Physiologie 1896;32:31–54.

[63] Feit J, Metelova M, Sindelka Z. Incorporation of 3H thymidine into damaged pulp of rat incisors. J Dent Res 1970;49(4):783–6.

[64] Fitzgerald M. Cellular mechanics of dentin bridge repair using 3H-thymidine. J Dent Res 1979;58(Spec Iss D):2198–206.

[65] Fitzgerald M, Chiego DJ Jr, Heys DR. Autoradiographic analysis of odontoblast replacement following pulp exposure in primate teeth. Arch Oral Biol 1990;35(9):707–15.

[66] Ruch JV. Patterned distribution of differentiating dental cells: facts and hypotheses. J Biol Buccale 1990;18(2):91–8.

[67] Ruch JV, Lesot H, Karcher-Djuricic V, et al. Facts and hypotheses concerning the control and differentiation. Differentiation 1982;21(1):7–12.

[68] Yamamura T. Differentiation of pulpal cells and inductive influences of various matrices with references to pulpal wound healing. J Dent Res 1985;64(Spec Iss):530–40.

[69] Goldberg M, Lasfargues JJ. Pulpo-dentinal complex revisited. J Dent Res 1995;23(1): 15–20.

[70] Ho AD. Kinetics and symmetry of divisions of hematopoietic stem cells. Exp Hematol 2005;33(1):1–8.

[71] Nakagawa H, Akita S, Fukui M, et al. Human mesenchymal stem cells successfully improve skin-substitute wound healing. Br J Dermatol 2005;153(1):29–36.

[72] Shi S, Bartold P, Miura M, et al. The efficacy of mesenchymal stem cells to regenerate and repair dental structures. Orthod Craniofac Res 2005;8(3):191–9.

[73] Rappel WJ, Thomas PJ, Levine H, et al. Establishing direction during chemotaxis in eukaryotic cells. Biophys J 2002;83(3):1361–7.

[74] Raftopoulou M, Hall A. Cell migration: Rho GTPases lead the way. Dev Biol 2004;265(1): 23–32.

[75] Weber DS, Taniyama Y, Rocic P, et al. Phosphoinositide-dependent kinase 1 and p21-activated protein kinase mediate reactive oxygen species-dependent regulation of platelet-derived growth factor-induced smooth muscle cell migration. Circ Res 2004;94(9):1219–26.

[76] Besson A, Gurian-West M, Schmidt A, et al. p27Kip1 modulates cell migration through the regulation of RhoA activation. Genes Dev 2004;18(8):862–76.

[77] Bach FH, Fineberg HV. Call for a moratorium on xenotransplants. Nature 1998; 22;391(6665)326.

[78] Hilton TJ. Cavity sealers, liners, and bases: current philosophies and indications for use. Oper Dent 1996;21(4):134–46.

[79] Brännstrom M, Lind PO. Pulpal response to early dental caries. J Dent Res 1965;44(5): 1045–50.

[80] About I, Murray PE, Franquin J-C, et al. Pulpal inflammatory responses following noncarious class V restorations. Oper Dent 2001;26(4):336–42.

[81] Bergenholtz G. Pathogenic mechanisms in pulpal disease. J Endod 1990;16(2):98–101.

[82] Murray PE, Smith AJ, Windsor LJ, et al. Remaining dentine thickness and human pulp responses. Int Endod J 2003;36(1):33–43.

[83] Donly KJ, Segura A, Kanellis M, et al. Clinical performance and caries inhibition of resin-modified glass ionomer cement and amalgam restorations. J Am Dent Assoc 1999;130(10): 1459–65.

[84] Maupome G, Sheiham A. Criteria for restoration replacement and restoration life-span estimates in an educational environment. J Oral Rehabil 1998;25(12):896–901.

[85] Burke FJ, Cheung SW, Mjör IA, et al. Reasons for the placement and replacement of restorations in vocational training practices. Prim Dent Care 1999;6(1):17–20.

[86] Dias WR, Pereira PN, Swift EJ Jr. Maximizing esthetic results in posterior restorations using composite opaquers. J Esthet Restor Dent 2001;13(4):219–27.

[87] Kelleher M, Bishop K. Tooth surface loss: an overview. Br Dent J 1999;186(2):61–6.

[88] Baran G, Boberick K, McCool J. Fatigue of restorative materials. Crit Rev Oral Biol Med 2001;12(4):350–60.

[89] Slavkin HC, Bringas P Jr, Bessem C, et al. Hertwig's epithelial root sheath differentiation and initial cementum and bone formation during long-term organ culture of mouse mandibular first molars using serumless, chemically-defined medium. J Periodontal Res 1989; 24(1):28–40.

[90] Thomas HF, Kollar EJ. Differentiation of odontoblasts in grafted recombinants of murine epithelial root sheath and dental mesenchyme. Arch Oral Biol 1989;34(1):27–35.

[91] Zeichner-David M, Diekwisch T, Fincham A, et al. Control of ameloblast differentiation. Int J Dev Biol 1995;39(1):69–92.

[92] Robey PG. Vertebrate mineralized matrix proteins: structure and function. Connect Tissue Res 1996;35(1–4):131–6.

[93] Wu D, Ikezawa K, Parker T, et al. Characterization of a collagenous cementum-derived attachment protein. J Bone Miner Res 1996;11(5):686–92.

[94] Bartlett JD, Simmer JP. Proteinases in developing dental enamel. Crit Rev Oral Biol Med 1999;10(4):425–41.

[95] Yamada M, Bringas P Jr, Grodin M, et al. Chemically-defined organ culture of embryonic tooth organs: morphogenesis, dentinogenesis, and amelogenesis. J Biol Buccale 1980;8(2): 127–39.

[96] Yoshikawa DK, Kollar EJ. Recombination experiments on the odontogenic roles of mouse dental papilla and dental sac tissues in ocular grafts. Arch Oral Biol 1981;26(4):303–7.

[97] Mina M, Kollar EJ. The induction of odontogenesis in a non-dental mesenchyme combined with early murine mandibular arch epithelium. Arch Oral Biol 1987;32(2):123–7.

[98] Choi RS, Vacanti JP. Preliminary studies of tissue-engineered intestine using isolated epithelial organoid units on tubular synthetic biodegradable scaffolds. Transplant Proc 1997; 29(1–2):848–51.

[99] Young CS, Terada S, Vacanti JP, et al. Tissue engineering of complex tooth structures on biodegradable polymer scaffolds. J Dent Res 2002;81(10):695–700.

[100] Kim SS, Vacanti JP. The current status of tissue engineering as potential therapy. Semin Pediatr Surg 1999;8(3):119–23.

[101] National Institute of Dental and Craniofacial Research. Biomimetics and tissue engineering. Bethesda (MD): National Institutes of Health; 2002.

[102] Tabak LA. Testimony before the House Subcommittee on Labor-HHS-Education Appropriations. March 28, 2001. Available at: http://www.hhs.gov/budget/testify/b20010516c.html. Accessed February 2, 2006.

ELSEVIER
SAUNDERS

Dent Clin N Am 50 (2006) 317–321

THE DENTAL
CLINICS
OF NORTH AMERICA

Index

Note: Page numbers of article titles are in **boldface** type.

dental.theclinics.com

Changing Your Address?

Make sure your subscription changes too! When you notify us of your new address, you can help make our job easier by including an exact copy of your Clinics label number with your old address (see illustration below.) This number identifies you to our computer system and will speed the processing of your address change. Please be sure this label number accompanies your old address and your corrected address—you can send an old Clinics label with your number on it or just copy it exactly and send it to the address listed below.

We appreciate your help in our attempt to give you continuous coverage. Thank you.

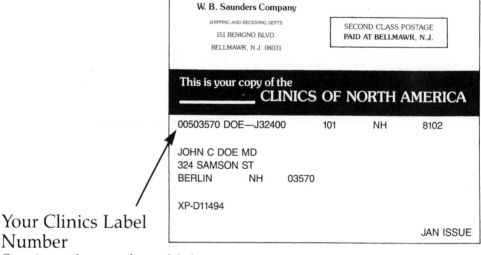

Your Clinics Label Number
Copy it exactly or send your label
along with your address to:
W.B. Saunders Company, Customer Service
Orlando, FL 32887-4800
Call Toll Free 1-800-654-2452

Please allow four to six weeks for delivery of new subscriptions and for processing address changes.